Creative D

# The Practice of Social Work
*General Editors: Bill Jordan and Jean Packman*

# Creative Day-Care

## For Mentally Handicapped People

### JAN CARTER

Basil Blackwell

Copyright © Jan Carter 1988
First published 1988

Basil Blackwell Ltd
108 Cowley Road, Oxford, OX4 1JF, UK

Basil Blackwell Inc.
432 Park Avenue South, Suite 1503
New York, NY 10016, USA

*British Library Cataloguing in Publication Data*

Carter, Jan
  Creative day care: for mentally handicapped
  people.—(The Practice of social work).
  1. Day care centres for the mentally handicapped
  I. Title    II. Series
  362.3′83              HV3004

ISBN 0–631–15519–8
ISBN 0–631–15731–X Pbk

*Library of Congress Cataloging in Publication Data*

Carter, Jan
  Creative day-care for mentally handicapped people.

  (The Practice of social work; 17)
  Bibliography: p.
  1. Day care centers for the mentally handicapped—
Great Britain—London.  2. Social work with the
mentally handicapped—Great Britain—London.  I. Title
II. Series.
HV3008.G7C37   1987        362.3′83        87–27647
ISBN 0–631–15519–8
ISBN 0–631–15731–X (pbk.)

Typeset in 11 on 12½ pt Times
by Opus, Oxford
Printed in Great Britain by Billing & Sons Ltd., Worcester

# Contents

For everything, there is a season, and a time . . .
a time to plant and a time to pluck . . .
a time to break down and a time to build up . . .

Ecclesiastes

# Preface

Too long
have we forgotten
that Peter and John and Eileen
– mentally deficient –
are people.

People who love and who want to be loved
who have joys
like you and me.
(You see we are normal people
. . . isn't it nice being normal?)

Peter and John and Eileen
have hearts that suffer
when we do not look at them
with respect
and love.

Too long have they been treated
like perpetual, dependent, incapable
children for whom we must do everything . . .

'Poor creatures,'
When will we learn,
When will we learn
that Peter and John and Eileen
have their rights for they are people
and more –
children of God.

We have too long despised them.
We have treated them with pitying
paternalism,
ignoring their potentialities.

We have forgotten
and they want
our respect
our love, but not smothering, protective love,
but love made up of esteem
and a desire to give life,
possibilities to create,
to give,
to feel useful to society.

They have a right to grow, to develop
in creativity and work
in joyful leisure,
in knowledge,
in small houses,
in spiritual life.

All these activities
should be open to them,
but we the so-called
normal people

(isn't it nice being normal . . . you and me?)

With atrophied hearts
and over-burdened minds,
obsessed by efficacity,
we forget that they are people . . .

From 'Too Long' by Jean Vanier

# Acknowledgements

This project was made possible by a grant from the Mental Health Foundation, London. It followed earlier work supported by the Joseph Rowntree Memorial Trust and the Department of Health and Social Security and reported in my book *Day Services for Adults: Somewhere to go (1981)*.

The staff and users of the Highbury Grove Centre in the London Borough of Islington supported this project with great interest and generosity. Special thanks and gratitude go to Christine Crowley.

Particular support and assistance at various points of the production of this book was given by Roy Parker, Grace Vaughan, Malcolm Williamson and Judyth Watson. The task of typing the manuscript was done with care by Dee Bourne (London) and Rene Nash (Perth).

Griffin House Graphics, Toronto are thanked for permission to reproduce part of Jean Vanier's poem 'Too Long', from *Eruption to Hope (1971)*.

Jan Carter

# Beginnings

## Purpose

This book is for those who are helping the people known as mentally or intellectually handicapped in the task of using time. It is directed, in the main, at the staff in day centres, hostels, workshops and hospitals and other recognized places of care, as well as to the unpaid volunteers and countless relatives and friends who are 'home' carers; those for whom the experience of living and working with a mentally handicapped person is a daily reality. But all concerned with quality of life for such persons, whether they are called mentally handicapped, mentally retarded, subnormal, slow learners, or intellectually deficient, may be interested in the experiences shared through this book.

For most of the past century, mentally handicapped girls and boys and men and women have been segregated into hospitals or hostels, or confined with their families and then forgotten. After the Second World War, activity programmes 'trained' mentally handicapped people to take on routine jobs in industry at the 'lower end' of the production section (Carter 1981). But in the 1970s and 1980s in Britain, manufacturing and production sectors of work shrank. Many working venues of care in social service or health agencies, such as hospital workshops or day training centres were unaware of these marked social changes. They have clung to their mission, to offer unskilled, but often exploited, labour to industries which in themselves have become less viable. Mentally handicapped people have been driven out of the job market and public policies have ignored the challenge: to devise new ways of living for groups of people who are excluded from long-term paid employment.

In the old days, it was of little importance to the majority of the community if time weighed heavily on the hands of those who were mentally handicapped, for they were viewed as an insignificant minority. Only about 240 people out of every 100,000 are severely mentally handicapped and roughly 2 per cent of the population are mildly mentally handicapped (Mittler 1979). These people could be thought to have nothing in common with the larger, more respectable majority. In the past, a few of the minority could always hope to achieve respectability, to become part of the majority. Occasionally, exceptions did 'make it' by getting and holding jobs. But the reduction in size of the full-time work-force led the definitions which asserted the difference between the minority and the majority to be redefined. The group outside the work-force and comprising the minority has not only been expanded but been complicated by the circumstances of poverty and social disadvantage (Mittler 1979).

It is not the purpose of this book to discuss definitions of mental handicap. But when compared with other major groups of persons outside the labour market, such as the elderly or racial minorities, more mentally handicapped persons are probably known to official agencies, and more are organized into services such as day centres or residential care. Thus mentally handicapped people are readily visible and because of this they are an ideal group with whom to raise the issue: how do they use their time?

The thread which runs through this book concerns the use of time. How to deal with time has become a recognized stress of the late twentieth century. One hundred and fifty years ago, the industrial revolution absorbed all available pairs of hands and nobody, with the possible exception of a small, favoured elite, worried about a surfeit of time. But compared with 150 years ago, declining numbers of people are now employed in full-time paid work and more people live longer into old age. And other handicapped persons, saved as infants and children by medical science, have survived into young adulthood. As unemployment rises and unskilled jobs in the manufacturing sector disappear, what are mentally or intellectually handicapped people to do with their time? Can our society offer more to mentally handicapped people than a life where they pass time, mark time, or merely 'do' time?

If mentally handicapped people continue to be blocked from entering the official labour market, how will the institutions catering for mentally handicapped people deal with long periods of time? In the past, institutions of all types have dealt with the passing of time by ignoring it. The calendar, not the clock, was the marker for those who lived in long-stay hospitals or for those who attended sheltered workshops. In these institutions every day was like most others. Certain inflexible routines marked out the major events of the day: washing, feeding, toileting, television. Perhaps church on Sunday morning and a club or a dance on Saturday night would vary these days from the rest. Walter, the man with Down's syndrome who is the hero of David Cook's novel *Winter Doves*, found when planning his escape from the mental handicap hospital that it was possible to predict exactly the behaviour and the movements of the staff and patients in the hospital at any minute of any hour of any day or night (Cook 1981).

Although this book discusses the use of time, it is neither abstract nor academic. The book's intention is practical, for it illustrates the use of time in one particular place: a day centre for mentally handicapped men and women. Although the book is not set in a residential institution, other places such as hospitals and hostels should be able to refer its approaches to their own situation.

That work with people in hospitals or institutions has important temporal features is not a new idea. The timing of the organization of work has been studied often, from the earliest time and motion men. More recently, Strauss and Glaser have argued that in hospitals the high incidence of death and the speed of dying affect the way nursing and other staff organize their work (Strauss and Glaser 1977). Similarly this book will suggest that the lower rates of discharge of mentally handicapped people from places of care and their slower responses to interventions have been matters which have affected the organization of their care too. The life-long nature of the handicap and the lifetime enrolment of most people in services has been associated with practices which might be described as either rigid and inflexible, or desultory, imprecise and laissez faire. Many of the practices are concerned less with developing the talents of users than in maintaining routines and rules for the staff. (See, for one analysis, Raynes, Pratt and Roses 1979.)

So this book is a case study in the temporal organization of care which will attempt to show that neither the rigid nor the desultory approaches are inevitable. The scene of the book is a day centre, and the script is a 'Monday-to-Friday' series. (Most day centres assemble on five days of each week.) The main actors are selected users and members of staff of the day centre – the Highbury Grove Adult Training Centre in North London – who speak for themselves about the way they use their time. They discuss in their own words the programmes they have devised, the activities which fill this, as opposed to that hour, the advantages and disadvantages of spending time at one activity compared with another. In addition the script of the day centre will be amplified by a narration. The narration will be drawn from the background to this project, information from a national survey of mentally handicapped persons attending day services in England and Wales (Carter 1981). Findings from this survey will be interpolated as and when they illuminate the activities of Highbury Grove Centre. The writer will assume the role of the narrator.

Until very recently, most medical and psychological texts about mentally handicapped persons have concentrated on defining their levels of mental function, or describing their deficits. The classifications which have emerged from this work have often, unwittingly, detracted from the fact that mentally handicapped people are, first and foremost, human. Although overtly antagonistic statements about them have become less common in the past decade, reduced discrimination in the community generally has not changed the ideologies of mental handicap still promoted in text-books. Few argue the case that mentally handicapped persons are like everyone else. Rather, most textbooks on mental handicap are about the differences which divide subnormal from normal.

The requirement of standards to divide normality from subnormality become less important when mentally handi-capped people are viewed as persons. Humans are, above all, individual; differences exist, in spite of levels of intelligence; variations are accepted in feelings, values and preferences. Mentally handicapped people, this book will show, are varied too. Their everyday circumstances affect their behaviour, shape their relationships and specify their preferences. Yet variation, a large part of what makes people human, is overlooked by most textbooks, which encourage the belief that mentally handicapped people can be standardized. This belief is very pervasive and one can trace its operation in everyday living by noting two particular strategies which stem from it.

First, the view that mentally handicapped people can be standardized implies that they are simply objects. As passive raw material, they wait, like blocks of marble, or stone, for a Great Sculptor (perhaps a doctor or a teacher) to fashion, painstakingly and slowly, a new creation, into a real human being. This approach considers that the main requirement for work with mentally handicapped people is to develop an appropriate set of behavioural techniques. The environment to which the techniques are applied is rarely considered, nor is the relationship between the Sculptor and the object or raw material. Perhaps Itard, who found the abandoned wild boy of Aveyron, Victor, and took him in to his house to train him, provides the classic example; it was the training, Itard considered, that led to Victor's limited progress (Lane 1977). It was not thought that either the environment Itard worked in, or his relationship with the boy had much impact. Itard was the classic Great Sculptor.

An alternative views the mentally handicapped person less as an inanimate object, than as a limited, unsocialized being, such as a credulous and limited child. Bernard Shaw's *Pygmalion* contrasts Professor Higgins, who is learned and omniscient, with Eliza Doolittle, who is a silly, backward woman. It is true that Eliza Doolittle does progress, but only as a result of the application of the Professor's superior expertise. Her 'improvements' are not due to ability on her part. Similarly, many writers see mentally handicapped people as 'tabula rasa', to be raised above the level of childhood. One well-known example is that of Amala and Kamala, two children found in a wolves' den in India at about ages one and eight (MacLean 1979). They were brought up by the Reverend Singh, the Indian priest who found them and tried desperately, but unsuccessfully, by example, to raise the children to his own level of table and other manners. When the children ignored his teachings he concluded that their unresponsiveness meant they were lesser human beings. They continued to walk on all fours and eat like wolves.

That mentally handicapped people are a separate category of being – either objects, or less than fully human – is an idea with a long history, which for centuries has justified their lifetime sentences of exclusion from society (Ryan 1980; Jones 1975). Even in the twentieth century, prominent social movements have rejected the right of mentally handicapped persons to marry. The eugenics school in the earlier decades of this century attempted to exclude mentally handicapped people from reproduction. Then later there were the chilling exterminations of mentally handicapped people by the Nazi regime. Both these discriminatory movements illustrate that mentally handicapped people can be viewed as less than fully human; they can be stripped automatically of the rights of personhood and citizenship.

Of course, not everyone who thinks that mentally handicapped persons are less-than-human would exterminate or sterilize them. Others may agree that they have no 'rights', but also take the softer line that precisely *because* they are less-than-human, mentally handicapped people have *needs* to which the more fortunate of us should minister. This belief has, in the past, justified the creation of venues of care away from the community. And the ideology that services should be based on needs rather than on rights is, perhaps, the key to understanding most current services, whether in health, education or social services.

In 'needs-based' services, mentally handicapped people can continue to be viewed as less-than-human by those who care for them. In this ethos, as we have seen, views about what constitutes progress are crucial. It will be argued that success is not sought by those who do not view the mentally handicapped as fully human, because it is rarely expected. This amplifies the pessimism which has become the corner-stone of many programmes. Pessimism about the lack of progress of a group such as the mentally handicapped is a powerful ideology. Its major value is that it keeps people in their places. It helps to maintain the traditional social order of a hospital, hostel or day centre. It does not disrupt the strict hierarchy in services, which insists that the helper maintain his or her dominance over the helped. It maintains that there are *some* who are less needy and more human than others (the staff), who help the *rest*, the very needy and less-than-human (in this case those with mental handicap).

There has been little consideration that progress in development by mentally handicapped people might be associated with matters *other* than the skills of the teacher, such as the type of *relationships* or the kind of *environment* in which the mentally handicapped person finds himself or herself. Yet in most other spheres, such as the home or the workplace, the quality of relationships and the calibre of the environment are crucial to development and progress. No-one thinks that a baby learns new skills solely because of his or her mother's skilful techniques. Certainly good techniques are helpful, but the *relationship* between mother and child and the everyday *setting* are central. It is helpful if the baby's learning takes place withn the context of an optimistic relationship, and within a benign and rewarding environment. And in the workplace, the type of relationship between worker and supervisor and the ambience of the office or factory affects the output.

These findings have not been applied seriously to mentally handicapped individuals. the types of human environments and personal relationships needed by mentally handicapped individuals to prosper have not been much studied. One exception is a study by Roy King, Norma Raynes and Jack Tizard, whose book *Patterns of Residential Care* showed that the everyday environment and type of relationships between staff and children were important. Small, decentralized units, where the staff had authority to take decisions and the flexibility to decide what programmes made for superior care were better for mentally handicapped children than large centralized institutions where staff were required to follow rigid routines and were told what to do (King, Raynes and Tizard 1971).

This supports the commonsense view that individuals, whether at home, at work, or even in care, get on best in those circumstances where they feel they are listened to and where they feel free to express themselves; in an environment which offers a sufficient degree of order for everyone to feel they have a role to play and a contribution to make to a common task. This is not to imply that techniques are not important. But good relationships and constructive working environments may be as important – if not more so – than precise techniques in the process of a mentally handicapped person acquiring a skill. This book will give the reader the chance to judge the relationships between techniques, environments and relationships.

Although the book will set out to discuss the use of time in a particular week in a particular place, the reader may like to consider some questions which come out of the chapters on the way through. First, there is the relationship between using time to develop a sense of COMPETENCE in mentally handicapped people. A particular approach to the use of time is necessary for users at the centre when compared with the rest of the world. Those we will meet do not fit the predetermined mould of the specific time in childhood provided for a standard education. So what are the special time frames for the development of competence for mentally handicapped people and how do staff apply this to their work? Does competence, as has been suggested, develop from certain relationships and particular types of environment?

Secondly, given that mentally handicapped people are slower and more laboured, are there circumstances where CREATIVITY shines through? Creativity is thought to be a gift of God (or of the gods) – an instantaneous flash of invention which is the mark of high intelligence and exceptional innovative ability. But is creativity to be associated only with speed, divine gifts and high intelligence? Or rather is it more a matter of application – the 'perspiration and inspiration' theory? And either way, given that they are slower and their timescales more elongated, are mentally handicapped people ever creative?

And thirdly, can a centre or an institution for the mentally handicapped become, over time, a real COMMUNITY? There have been many efforts by scholars and reformers to specify the features of communal living in the past two decades, but with some notable exceptions (such as the L'Arche movement), little of this enthusiasm has affected the institutions of mental handicap. Mostly life in the long-term institution is viewed as a sentence. Yet could it be that an enclosed community where few people ever leave *might* also become a setting where a healing community might flourish? The success of such communities stands or falls by the quality of relationships of the inhabitants. So can long-term supportive communities, on a day or residential basis, be established in a setting where most people are mentally handicapped?

## Place

The experiences reported in this book come from a day centre in North London, the Highbury Grove Centre in the London Borough of Islington. For a month in a recent summer, people at the Centre were questioned, observed, tape-recorded and timed, in an effort to understand *why* the Centre ran the way it did, *what* the staff were trying to do and *how* they went about their job. What emerged from these discussions forms the main part of the book, the chapters 'Monday' to 'Friday'. These describe a day in the life of some of the Centre's users and some staff. The use of time to get through the day – whether the seven-hour day of the Centre; the sixteen-hour day of the hostel, or the twenty-four hours of the hospital is a major preoccupation. So the time of the day will be reflected by dealing, in turn, with a day of the week, from Monday to Friday.

Why was Highbury Grove, the centre of all this activity, chosen as the site for the book? Along with dozens of other day centres, Highbury Grove Centre has taken part in a national survey of day care during the mid-1970s. A major research project had surveyed the varying types of day care in England and Wales and eventually located 290 day units in a census taken in 13 areas of England and Wales. Of these, 50 units were training centres (as they were then called) for people with mental handicap. The project interviewed 105 staff and 193 users in training centres for mentally handicapped people across the country. Their opinions are recorded elsewhere (Carter 1981). Most training or day centres were dull, apathetic and unimaginative places. Highbury Grove Centre, the subject of this book was an exception.

For many years, Highbury Grove had been a traditional mental handicap training centre. It offered a contract work programme which concentrated exclusively on giving users routine tasks such as packing envelopes into boxes, month by month, year by year. Token gestures to the necessity for further education, (particularly reading and writing) were restricted by the lack of space. But the staff and users began to question their philosophy and their programme at the time they were planning to move into a new building. Now, five years later, the staff and users of Highbury Grove are able to tell the story of what had happened in the intervening years and how changes had affected its staff and its 70 or so users, aged from 16 to 60 years.

Today, Highbury Grove Centre, in a tree-lined street in North London's Islington, looks anonymous and slightly shabby. Its plain brick and glass single storey could suggest a clinic, a school, or perhaps a small factory. A narrow frontage gives on to the street, but inside, a labyrinth of corridors and spaces confuses the visitor. There are large spaces, such as a hall-cum-dining room and a gym, and small spaces such as workrooms, classrooms and a library. There are inside spaces and outside spaces. There are streams of people busily heading to classroom or craftroom in pursuit of activities which appear complicated and difficult to grasp. It is very different to the simple, ordered layout of a hospital ward, or a workshop.

Highbury Grove has developed from a very simple organization, where everyone did the same work at the same time, to a complex organization where nearly everybody, the 70 users and the 15 staff, is doing something different at the same point in time. The change in complexity of the time sequences is one of the key points to understanding this Centre and the story of change in this book. How have the activities altered? How was the work programme scrapped? How has education become the *raison d'être* of the Centre? How have staff and users developed new roles and different kinds of relationships?

Each user of the Centre has an individually tailored timetable to take him or her through the week. So the Centre has swung from the old demand that the user fit into the Centre's programme to the new attempt to make the Centre fit each of the 70 or so users.

Five years ago Highbury Grove could be described as

rigid, unimaginative, dull. It retained many of the negative aspects of the hospital it had set out to replace. It was good for filling in time by keeping mentally handicapped people off the streets during the day, and it was efficient at offering their families 'time out'. The staff had pronounced views on the importance of 'developing full potential' or 'achieving independence' for their users, but there was little evidence that this rhetoric was put into action.

The old Highbury Grove was not an isolated case. It is important to reconsider the role of such centres; the reality is that very few users ever leave, or are likely to leave day centres to take up jobs. In fact, almost all the users of such centres can expect to stay for the rest of their lives (Carter 1981). In the future it may become more and more difficult to find a place in a centre such as Highbury Grove. So how can the day centres of today avoid becoming the warehouses of tomorrow, taking their place alongside, or replacing the long-stay hospitals as the ghettos of the future?

This book sets out to show that a day centre can be more than a warehouse. But it has the problem that the 70 or so programmes for each of the users at Highbury Grove cannot be collapsed into one small book. To compromise, from Monday through to Friday, we will, each day, meet a selected user of Highbury Grove Centre and his or her particular staff members, who will outline the way they spend their time. On *Monday*, the user in question will be one of the more disabled members of the Centre, Leanne, who is as dependent on the Centre as any user. She needs to be fed, to be dressed, to be toileted. Nor can she speak, although she can walk. But by the time we reach Friday, the user is as independent as Leanne is dependent. Samantha, born with Down's syndrome, is an articulate member of the Centre. She has a part-time volunteer job; sings in a rock group and wants to leave her parent's home to get a flat. In the future, she would love to be completely independent of the Centre.

Between, on Tuesday, Wednesday and Thursday, we meet Clive, Paul and Dee. But there is little point in introducing these users and their individual programmes on their own. It is as important to discuss the tasks and the role of the staff, the kind of environment the staff and users create, the relationships they forge, and the skills the staff use. The job of staff with mentally handicapped people is sometimes summed up in phrases such as 'promoting independence', 'developing full potential' or achieving 'social acceptability'. What do these phrases mean and, above all, what does one actually do to achieve them? What practical steps are involved in achieving social acceptability or independence? The staff will try to explain these matters in their own words.

So this book will introduce a mosaic of activities used to structure time with mentally handicapped people, whilst, at the same time, describing the job of the staff and trying to show how all these activities mesh together in one organization. For example, to get through a week, a user needs to thread himself or herself through a complicated building and complex programme. He or she may spend part or all of the time assigned to one of the three 'majors' in the Centre in the unit known as Special Needs, at the Education department or in the Arts and Crafts department. Each of these 'majors' is then subdivided into specific group activities. Thus, Arts and Crafts includes pottery, painting, drawing and printing; whilst Education covers literacy, numeracy, cooking, drama, shopping and travel (amongst other things). At first, the reader may find it hard to distinguish the logic behind the programmes, so that passing time on 'Monday' may be as complex for the reader as it is for a new staff member. But, given time, by 'Friday' the principles of planning time for mentally handicapped individuals should be clear.

In examining issues related to competence, creativity and community within a day centre, this book will also argue that most mentally or intellectually handicapped people are exposed to a future where they will continue to be excluded from traditional, paid jobs. This generalization is not meant to detract from efforts to create innovative work programmes or work schemes, nor is it intended to deter staff in centres from strenuous efforts in trying to place individuals in jobs.

Indeed, the book suggests that more resources be devoted to work support schemes, so that more mentally handicapped people are supported through their entry to and consolidation in the work-force. However, while acknowledging that efforts need to be made to find jobs for mentally handicapped people, the book also challenges the assumption that the only way for mentally handicapped people to achieve a fulfilled life is through a paid job. It is true that our society places a high status on participation in the work-force and that there is an association between personal feelings of work and self esteem, being able to escape from poverty and having a job. But to hold out the future promise of paid work to most mentally handicapped people in the 1980s would be futile. Encouragement to develop confidence in personal competence, participation in a community where the individual is valued and respected, opportunity to express oneself creatively and develop new skills are all possibilities which this book will seek to amplify.

# Monday

## Who's Who on Monday

*Leanne* is the focus of today's events. She is a severely mentally handicapped young woman, in late teenage. Although able to walk, she depends on others completely for her food, dressing and toileting. She loves people and jogging and is gregarious and energetic.

*Cathy* is the staff member with special responsibilities for Leanne in particular and the multiply handicapped, or 'Special Needs', users in general. A graduate in psychology, she is in her mid-twenties and attractive, brisk and purposeful in movement and manner.

*Philippa* is a care assistant and has worked at the Centre for about six months. Tall, friendly and thoughtful in manner, she has a gentle certainty and confidence about her approach to her work. She is a graduate and has worked for a time in a mental hospital.

*Tom* is a profoundly mentally handicapped young man from a West Indian family. He has a sweet and loving disposition and he enjoys touching people, a trait not always easy for others to accept.

*Rita* is confined to a wheelchair and is very deaf, as well as suffering from poor sight. Her manner is dour and uncompromising, but she can apply her hands to a task with surprising speed.

*Godfrey* is a mystery. He has strange habits, known officially as behavioural disorders. He is feared for his unpredictable moods and movements and has been called autistic.

*Jo* is on the staff, a care assistant with a sweet manner and engaging smile. She is reliable and painstaking at her work.

*Mitch* is a visiting drama teacher, who has another life as a clown. He visits the Centre on Mondays.
*Anil* is co-leader, with Cathy, of the Special Needs Unit. He is also the Centre's music specialist – because (he says modestly) he at least plays the piano badly. He is a former mathematician and computer person.


9.00 Introduction

London. A heavy summer's morning. Schoolboys on bicycles dart between motorists. Motorists weave between red buses. Red buses snake between thundering lorries. From this patterned chaos emerges a white coach, which hoots its way onto a shallow forecourt in front of a modest brick and glass building. The coach shudders to a stop. There is a momentary silence. Passengers appear. Mostly young people, they spill onto the forecourt and are swallowed inside the plate-glass door, kept private by the sun's reflections on the glass.

A young woman emerges, aged about 25 and dressed in trousers with casual cotton sweater. She looks as if she is off to play tennis. She enters the bus and then shepherds off a younger woman, dumpy, dressed in a summer floral print dress. They lurch through the plate-glass door, as the younger woman makes friendly roaring noises. The youngish woman with the tennis image, Cathy, has her arm around the noisy woman in the print dress, Leanne. Arms interlocked, they make a slow bumpy progress along a narrow corridor, Leanne lurching sideways into the walls. Eventually, the procession reaches a door marked 'Special Needs' and enters – a large, airy room with French windows leading onto a small unmade garden. The room itself is a friendly clutter. On low cupboards standing against the wall, there is a record player, books, magazines, plants, china and cutlery. There are children's games, painting equipment, musical instruments such as gongs, cymbals, and a set of drums. In the middle is a group of noisy people, mostly young, obviously handicapped, sitting in a circle. A tall young woman moves to the piano. The morning is about to begin.

Today, Monday, we will follow some of the work of some members of the Special Needs Unit. Collected from home or hostel by the coach, they will spend the day at the Centre. First, we talk to Cathy, the special care worker about the aims and methods of making up a weekly programme to meet Leanne's particular problems and needs. Second, we watch a teaching session with blind Tom. What is the Centre trying to achieve with his fey nature? Third, Rita, who is deaf, spends an hour on the loo, supervised by Philippa. Fourth, we go to a drama group with Godfrey; and finally, end with music.

## 9.05 Special Needs Care Group

*Cathy* 'Special Needs' meet Monday to Friday in this room, set apart from the rest of the Centre. There are ten people in the group, each with two or more handicaps such as blindness, deafness or immobility, but one constant handicap, mental retardation. First thing each morning, small groups of five or six users meet at the same spot with a particular staff member who ensures their personal care. I have five Special Needs users including Leanne.

As a care worker I'm responsible for her social and medical care. It's my job to do liaison work with her parents and with others who may be in touch with her. I keep account of her files and prepare her annual review. After the reviews I'm responsible for carrying through new developments into her programme. It's surprising how much work this involves, even for only five people.

Leanne is severely mentally handicapped. She has no speech, but she makes loud screaming noises – frequently! She's incontinent, so toileting is the main part of her programme. For four months we marked off her chart every time she was toileted; whether she was dry or wet. Then, with our psychologist, we looked at the results and worked out new times for toilet sessions. At the moment, she goes to the toilet seven times a day, on every hour, which is quite a lot. But she actually sometimes takes herself now; once she's there she knows what to do. So that's progress. The long-term aim is for her to be able to go herself.

Second, we're trying to lengthen her attention and concentration which is very limited. She likes water, and food. So for play, we concentrate on food and water materials.

A third priority is exercise. She's short and quite plump, so she does sport and goes jogging. A play session in the play room to help her to use up physical energy. She goes to gardening and gets exercise there.

Fourth, she gets a lot out of music. She made a musical instrument for herself. It's wooden sticks, painted. They hang on a bar, like a chime bar. She can hit them, or knock them together in music sessions, so she can actually see the end result.

Fifth, she also does craft and she's made a plaster of Paris model. The end result wasn't very amazing, but she enjoyed getting her hands dirty. If we can make it seem like play for Leanne, we can win her attention much more easily. So that's her week here.

### Leanne's Programme

| | Today is *Monday* | *Tuesday* | *Wednesday* | *Thursday* | *Friday* |
|---|---|---|---|---|---|
| AM | Gardening | Craft | Social training | Gardening | Physical therapy, therapy & jogging |
| PM | Music | Play | Free | Craft | Free choice |

Toilet at 9.00, 10.30, 11.30, 1.00, 2.00, 3.00 and 3.45

NO DRINK AFTER LUNCH

## 9.30 Activities

The 'Special Needers' are nearly all under 30 and their handicaps include blindness, deafness and spasticity. While half the group are confined to wheelchairs, the rest are mobile 'dashers'. So there are physical demands in working with people who need either to be pushed and lifted, or restrained and dampened down.

The dour Rita is aged about 25. Lopsided in her wheelchair, she is also profoundly deaf, with very limited vision. With these disabilities, her mental competence has been difficult to assess. At present she is efficient and accurate. Cathy praises her. She tells me that Rita's father – an immigrant single parent – speaks only limited English. Rita is an example of the way that a label of mental handicap can be shaped by many factors extraneous to intelligence: lack of hearing, poor sight and a non-English-speaking environment.

By contrast there is effervescent, warm Tom. But compared with Rita, Tom's concentration is poor and he can only attend for about 20 minutes at a time. Cathy takes Tom to the cupboard to teach him the difference between 'on' and 'in'. He feels five familiar objects (cup, spoon, fork, knife, plate) all over. Cathy shows him the top of the cupboard and then inside.

'Put the *fork on* the cupboard, Tom!'

'Put the *cup in* the cupboard, Tom!'

Unlike most of the Special Needs users, Tom has a few gutteral words: – 'Fork,' he barks. 'Cup . . . in cupboard.' He will practise this task four or five times today. When Cathy takes Tom to the Arts and Crafts room this afternoon she will explain this exercise to the craft instructor, so that Tom uses this exercise by putting his paint brush *on*, or *in* the sink.

## 10.30 Break

The staff move with the 'Special Needs' people to the dining room for coffee. Getting Leanne, Tom, Rita, Godfrey and the others there is time-consuming and tiring. Unlike the rest of the users of the Centre, those in the Special Needs group do not queue at the counter for drinks: they are given their food at the table. Soon the table tops are awash with coffee, milk and broken biscuits. The other users sit at laminate-covered tables for four, and the staff group around two tables.

Cathy continues to talk about the way the Special Needs group is organized. Other day centres segregate the Special Needs users from the rest so that staff who work with the multiply handicapped are isolated from the rest of the Centre and its way of life. How does this centre deal with the problem?

*Cathy*  First, we have a good ratio of staff to users. If our ratio was bad there'd be a bit to moan about. But six staff to ten users is good. The ratio is particularly important: with the Special Needs group you can't set up what we call 'holding' activities as you can with the rest (when we put a group to work on a task so that we can concentrate on one or two, doing something more specific). But with the multiply handicapped who need more, not less supervision, a higher staff ratio is crucial. Otherwise you're just 'containing' someone like Leanne, not working with her.

Second, the other factor that helps the integration between Special Needs and the rest of the Centre is joint activities. We use the Special Needs room mainly as a 'base' for scheduled activites like music or education, for any seven users at a time. But at any one time, about three users go out from the 'base' into the rest of the Centre. Leanne is to go jogging with Jo later. Godfrey and Leanne will go to drama this afternoon with me. Some users from the rest of the Centre will come in here for an activity. For example, two come into the cooking group.

Third, other staff from the Centre come in to teach the Special Needs users. Two run physical therapy sessions; another specializes in remedial education. That helps the integration of the multiply handicapped users with the rest of the Centre. It's a two-way thing, we're not just 'us' and 'them'.

Yes, a centre that isolated the Special Needs people so that staff only worked with people like Leanne could get really depressing. In the rest of the Centre, you can, at least, aim towards an end. But for users with multiple handicaps, the actual *value* of an activity isn't always the *result*. It's the *doing* it. Take cooking. You can't expect Leanne to make her own tea, or snack, whereas with some other users in the Centre you can. For Leanne it can be demoralizing just to stop and think, 'What aim am I achieving?' You have to look at it quite differently. A lot of our programme is aimed towards the end of providing more stimulation; to extending attention and concentration. It applies in the rest of the Centre, but probably more so here. You could get a bit 'down' if you started thinking about end results.

## 11.00 Hygiene

I am invited by Philippa to share a toileting session for Rita. This large woman weighs thirteen stone; there is a lot of heaving and panting in getting her from wheelchair to toilet. Why take the trouble, I ask?

*Philippa* First, we're trying to help Rita with showering each week, because her father is on his own and finds it difficult to cope as she's so heavy! Second, we're starting to try to get her to help undress herself. But the biggest thing of all with Rita is the toilet. We're training her to go regularly so that she'll become continent. Six months ago, we used to lift her up, but now she *can* stand herself up and usually she holds on to the rails while we pull her trousers down. Then she moves sideways and sits herself down. And the biggest thing so far is that she can now sit herself back in her wheelchair.

Now, *that* fits in with her programme because at physio-therapy she pulls herself up from sitting positions, steps sideways to separate her limbs and sits down. That means that every day she goes to the toilet – and gets her physio exercises as well. But she needs such a lot of encouragement! She gets a bit uptight and *screams* if she's doing something she doesn't like. When we were teaching her to go to the toilet, she was so nervous. When she got flustered, she'd scream and scream and scream. She's very, very limited in what she communicates: at home she can point to the commode when she wants the toilet but that's all.

We take her to the toilet after break, and after dinner every day. She takes ages! She has to be left on for twenty minutes or so, like now. Sometimes she doesn't want to go and when it's her period she hates it, because it confuses her signals that she wants to go to the loo early. If she wets it's just when her period starts. That's what I've noticed, anyway.

[We are faced by a wait: I change the subject. Why is a university graduate like Philippa spending her days toileting handicapped people?]

After I had finished my degree, I worked in a mental hospital. It wasn't a good set-up and compared to this Centre, it was really bad. I was on a ward with severely mentally handicapped adult women and there was nothing like getting them to help themselves. The attitude was that they were there because they *couldn't* help themselves. Our job was to feed them and wash them. If Rita were there she would just be plonked on the toilet, taken off an hour later, plonked back into the ward, in some corner. The staff would get on with their jobs. At tea-time, she'd be fed again, dumped in a bath and put into bed. That was the day, constant feeding and watering. You never actually helped anyone to help themselves, because that wasn't what *you* were there for and that wasn't what *they* were there for. 'They can't do anything . . . so what's the use in trying?'

If Rita were there, she wouldn't have been considered a *person* with any form of *preferences*, really. She would have been thought dumb. But Rita does have preferences. She *does* enjoy things and she *does* like doing things for herself. She responds to encouragement. Okay, Rita's very limited but you can bring her forward. In the hospital, problems like smearing or bad behaviour or sexual problems were common. You *never see* them here. Ellen stood in the same corner every day rocking for seventeen years. On the same floor, in the same hospital. and no-one ever bothered to try anything. It wasn't that the staff were really *callous* . . . You come on at half seven in the mornings and you don't finish until eight o'clock at night. You've got seventeen people (some with really difficult behaviour problems) and three staff. Most time is spent washing, feeding, changing. 'In-out, in-out, in-out.' Undress, bathe, dry, put on dressing gown, shove them back in the ward, lock the door so they can't get out while you are in the bathroom with the next one.

It was partly a staff shortage, but I think it was just the whole attitude towards mental hospitals. This one was viewed as a dustbin. There's nowhere else, so you just stick people in a hospital. Some staff were really caring but the situation is self-perpetuating. No-one ever tried. The low pay justified the lack of use of trying. And the majority of jobs were *very* heavy. Floors to be kept clean, chairs to be kept clean, beds to keep clean.

But here, I'm *doing* something. I get results. And I'm working with '*people*' rather than the 'mentally handicap-ped'. In the hospital we were admired by outsiders: 'Oh I just couldn't do that!' The mentally handicapped were thought to be ogres and in some ways you felt you were being a martyr. But here you don't get that. You're working with *people*, people with differences and their own opinions. You help them to do those things they need help with.

People here look happier, they look better, they're all dressed nicely. Here, as staff, you're not just the maid cleaning a machine, or keeping a body in working order – you're doing things with people. Really, at the hospital, all we did was to take clothes on and off, bathe and wash. If you spent time with your patients, you got on the wrong side of the senior staff, because that 'wasn't the done thing'. I was a lot harder on patients than I am here. It was almost expected of you, that's the way it was done.

## 12.00 Jogging

A special jogging session has been arranged for Leanne. Accompanied by Jo, we change into our blue and green track suits in the washrooms. Leanne roars with prospective pleasure and lurches very fast down the corridor, out through the plate-glass front door. We restrain her across the busy road, into the park. Once outside the Centre, Leanne's lion noises stop. Her lurching because sedate: according to Jo, Leanne is very 'good' when she is out of the Centre. Leanne can move fast: it is quite an effort for the better co-ordinated, but chatting, pair of us to keep up.

There are few people in the park. It is not school holidays and rather too early for the lunch-time spill from nearby offices. Jo tells me that Leanne often attracts curious glances from the local joggers: relations between the public and the users of the Centre are frequently uneasy. By now we have run the length of the elongated park – more of a green really – and Jo and I are being outpaced. On the return lap, Jo explains the point of Leanne's exercise programme.

*Jo*  Leanne gets a lot out of sports, more than some of the others, because she loves company so much. She really does relate to the more able clients who are very motherly and fatherly towards her. And they praise her, which she adores. She absolutely loves the praise she gets at the end of a race. She's rushed around (obviously with help) and they cheer her when she comes in. She really reacts to that: her face lights up. At first she never really joined in. She didn't use to do exercises, simply because it just wasn't in her personality to wave her arms about and lift her legs up and down. But in competitive things like ball games, obstacle races and netball, with encouragement, she shows enthusiasm. *And* she loves jogging. If you encourage her, she'll run anywhere

Leanne's very good when she's 'out', she never misbehaves. She has really marvellous behaviour in public. She knows that she just mustn't shriek. She runs around the

Centre shrieking at the top of her voice, but when she's out she almost never shouts or cries, even when she's really excited.

## 12.30 Lunch

At lunch, Leanne shrieks happily into the steak and kidney pudding, fed to her by Jo. Next year, Jo says, the plan is to begin to teach Leanne to feed herself. Philippa reports that Rita has helped herself into her chair voluntarily twice running. Tom spills his coffee over the table and Jo's skirt. Godfrey sits at a table on his own and glowers at a ham salad. Leanne's cheerful roaring can be heard above the noise level of the 70 or so people in the hall. A stranger joins the table and introduces himself as Mitch, the visiting drama teacher, quiet and ascetic and with a serious manner. He explains, improbably, that he works as a clown.

Whereas morning in the Centre is usually a two-session affair, the afternoon is normally unbroken, except for a cup of tea. But since the Special Needs folk have short attention spans, their time is often organized rather differently. For most of the group, the afternoon will be spent at music-making in their base room, with Anil, the Centre's music man. But early in the afternoon two of the Special Needers, Godfrey and Leanne, will join the drama group.

*Jo* This afternoon I'm going to work with Leanne and Godfrey. He's got quite extreme behaviour problems, as you might have noticed. You will meet him at drama, so I'll explain in advance. He sits shredding newspaper all day. He sits on the heater in his own corner, the only place he feels safe. He doesn't interact with others at all, partly because he is deaf. So on Monday afternoons I take Godfrey into the drama group. Just very briefly, just for as long as Godfrey will tolerate; then we go on to craft. But it does him good to be with other people and to get him out of the Special Needs room . . . Different faces, nice big room, new room, different room. But when I'm with Godfrey I've got to work with him solidly, or I'll find someone else on the floor after

Godfrey has thumped them. I can't leave him for a second, whereas I can leave Leanne, she's so easy-going.

We haven't sent Leanne to drama until recently but at present she is getting such a lot out of relating to each other that we've decided she should join us too. My own work is very spread out: through the week I work with every individual in the Special Needs group. The care assistants share the same duties as instructors like Cathy, but although we are supposed to do more of the physical tasks, in our Centre, it's shared. I wouldn't do any more toileting than Cathy, for example, because we work with people rather than tasks.

## 2.00 Drama

Lunch has finished. Some users sit together, a few play table tennis, several hold hands, but most just sit alone without much interest in surroundings. Towards two o'clock, there is an exodus from the dining hall as people gradually drift towards the afternoon activities held in about eight separate rooms. The Monday drama session is mounted for a selected group, chosen because of difficulties in communicating with staff and each other. This group is drawn from the Centre as a whole, with two participants today, Godfrey and Leanne, drawn from Special Needs.

The drama group meets in a small hall in the Centre, used as a gym. We (minus Godfrey and Leanne) stand in a circle, hands joined. We draw circles, in turn, with our hands and elbows, our feet and necks. The door opens. Jo almost falls through with a reluctant Godfrey and grinning Leanne. They join the circle. Godfrey draws awkward cicles with his hands and feet on request. But he grows restive quickly and Jo takes him out, leaving Leanne. At least Godfrey's time with the drama group has increased: on his first day, eight weeks ago, he stayed ten seconds! Today's length was three minutes.

Circles in the air become more extravagant: Leanne's require direction. Mitch introduces today's play. We are at a circus. First, an instrument parade. Everyone plays a chosen instrument. Leanne loves joining in. Oompha, oompha, oompha, here comes the band: drums, trumpets, percussion, a clarinet. Next the circus acts. Two clowns followed by a ballerina, a juggler, lions, a gorilla and a high trapeze act march in. The band and the acts rehearse for the 'real' performance, from Grand Parade to Finale. Everyone has an act, choreographed by Mitch. My lion tamer act draws admiration from my new friends. Was I really a teacher, or a student, asks Peta? Finally, Mitch plays music for the circus animals, people and musicians to join in a grand dance. Leanne is very, very happy. The circus dissolves as the group leave the room cackling with laughter and wheezing with good humour. I ask Mitch to explain his work.

*Mitch* I use mime to develop non-verbal communication skills. We discuss what we're doing, too, so altogether we use the body, the voice and feelings.

Today was a usual day. We had a light warm-up to move parts of the body, to create a sense of body awareness and to loosen up. It enabled even Leanne and Godfrey to work with us at the beginning. It's interesting to ask them for a movement each. I say, 'You do a movement and we'll all copy.' From their point of view, it gives a chance for initiative and it promotes a group feeling, throughout. So that's what 'warm-up' is about.

The circus was part of a sequence: we've been acting out a series of stories. The content is usually a fairytale which gives an opportunity for relating to each other. Last week was a very simple example. First we did some musical mime; all playing a different 'instrument' . . . guitar, trombone, piano . . . as we did today. *I* was an old man who liked music, but could never hear music in my house. *They* were people who played music, but never had anyone to play to. The old man opens his upstairs window . . . and the musicians open theirs. The old man hears music . . . and *he* is happy. The musicians play music . . . and *they* are happy. So they played louder and louder! And then I used a record which has sentiments about music making you feel cheerful. From that, we went on to act out simple feelings – being happy, being sad, being proud. To follow I made up a story called 'The Clown that Doesn't Smile'. A clown woke up in the morning and couldn't smile. We invented ways in which the clown found his smile . . .

Perhaps next week we'll do another story called 'The Wish'. A group of people will go for a walk and discover a bird with a broken wing, in a tree. They'll take the bird down and feed it. Then the bird will fly away and turn into a magician, who rewards everybody for their kindness, with a wish. They will sit down and share their individual wishes with each other. To be a juggler? A yo-yo? A flower? There are certain caring things (like taking the bird down and feeding it), which reverse the role of them being the people cared for all the time. It gives them the feeling of sharing and taking responsibility towards somebody else.

Sometimes we sit down, and finish off with a mime of something each person did yesterday. 'Yesterday', on Mondays, is Sunday, and usually a recreational day. Or I say: 'Do a mime of something you're going to do tomorrow.' Just simple requests recalling 'yesterday' demands concentration and memory. Then we finish off with a dance. It's a varied group. The main limit is lack of comprehension. Sometimes there may be an emotional impediment as well, as for instance with Godfrey. He is a very sweet person but he gets quite angry and is moody. But the plusses are that the *group* is good-natured and responsive. They are open and candid and quite imaginative. Some have natural aptitude. Watching Theresa today do an absolutely beautiful mime, with flowing movements. What she was doing was apparent to an onlooker.

A lot of it is educating latent qualities: if you're asking for a mime their response would be as imaginative as anybody else's. There's also a lot of humour in the group and that's good to work with comprehension, so the group has developed an imagination, a group awareness, and an ability to articulate. Their confidence to do all that has increased over time.

Sometimes they imitate me, or something they've seen before. But that's not bad; it demonstrates my relationship with them. The group is physically and imaginatively quite demanding, so it is paced to an hour and a half. Otherwise restlessness might set in. But this is a more benign and more openly responsive group than I find at the psychiatric centre where I also work. Most art forms are very good for mentally handicapped people. Anything that encourages their sensibilities, rather than aggressive attitudes. A mixture of different artists and therapists should work together. There should be music, dance, drama, movement, mime, art therapy, object makers. This Centre has the beginning of this.

## 3.00 Music

We are interrupted by the afternoon tea trolley known colloquially as 'Shop'. Tea, cold drinks, biscuits and cakes are sold by rostered users, who buy their goods at local shops in the morning and sell them in the afternoon. At the Special Needs base, the music group is assembled. Most participants have been there since the lunch break. Anil conducts. He is a Sri Lankan-born, British-educated maths graduate. He plays the piano – Percy Grainger's 'Country Garden' while each 'Special Needer' plays a simple instrument. There are drums, tambourines, sticks and chimes. This strange music circle is ignored by Godfrey, safely back on his corner heater after his exposure to the wider world. Leanne has had a good day and she beats her chime bar vigorously, if at random. Tom is trying to clutch Jo, who is trying to get him to clutch a tambourine. Rita is slumped over a drumstick. Philippa leads the singing (by staff) of 'When the Saints Go Marching In'. At any one point of time about half the Special Needers seem attentive. Leaving the group to Philippa, Anil moves aside to tell me about the music group.

*Anil* Special Needs are not so much a group as a set of individuals. There's no real group identity: they're so profoundly handicapped that they don't relate to each other much. So first, music tends to be a unifier, a group activity. We're concentrating on playing together, as a group. Very difficult! Sometimes we don't have the whole group playing together, only four or five . . . But at the end of Monday we *have* done something together as a *group*, rather than as *individuals* . . .

Second, rhythm is a very strong instinct in most mentally handicapped people, so we concentrate on rhythm to work on gross motor movements. For example, using rhythm to beat the drum or click a tambourine. When people don't respond to any rhythm impulses at all, you are, in a sense, lost.

We have banging sessions. For ten minutes we just bang the drum – as one group, one drum. Suddenly, someone who you'd never dream would pick up a drumstick, let alone play it, will suddenly do just that, pick it up off the floor and actually bang a drum. (Little things like that are fantastic breakthroughs.) You snatch on that, leave everybody else, zoom in on that person . . . (generally that's a mistake because they withdraw). But you have times where you're lifted seven feet off the floor! So we emphasize the *group process* and the *rhythm* aspects of music.

A third technique is to listen. Last week the other group in the Centre played Mussorgsky's 'Night on a Bare Mountain', on record. That piece of music is good for listening, because it is dramatic, with pictures to work on – the idea of spending a night on a bare mountain. So listening is thinking about it, evoking a picture of it, acting out the scene. People shut their eyes to imagine themselves alone on a bare mountain. Think what they would feel! Hungry, cold and frightened. We would see dinosaurs, snakes, the moon, stars, lightning and thunder!

After listening, we act our story by playing a set of tunnel drums, chime bars, and the usual percussion stuff – tambourine, sticks (which are basically just sticks of dowel).

That's about all, at present (money's the problem). We need more wind instruments, things like penny whistles.

So music is a medium for interaction, rhythm, listening and playing. But we try to develop other skills. Co-ordination and concentration. Even banging a drum for ten minutes for Leanne demands both those.

You asked me how I came to be working at music here? Well it's relevant to this. I'd done a maths degree, then I was a computer programmer for about four years, before that became boring – not in terms of the work I was doing, but unstimulating in the rewards. The main reward was money and the excitement of problem solving, which was OK but very abstract.

It struck me that problem solving could be applied in working with people. I had a vague wishy-washy idea that I wanted to go into the caring professions, a semi-noble sentiment, I suppose. I worked for a time, for about six months, in the local mental handicap hospital, one of those cut off from the community, in peaceful sourroundings in Surrey. I could see the potential: when volunteers came in from the outside, it seemed the one ray of sunshine. The rest of the time they were sitting about doing nothing.

In a way, you've got to have a more human relationship with mentally handicapped people than with any other group. If you don't, you end up treating them like machines, or pet animals, or small children. You have to bear in mind constantly that they are adult human beings like yourself. It is very tempting to opt for the pet, or even the small child relationship, with the Special Needs group especially because they are, in so many ways, like children. This is the biggest problem in working with mentally handicapped people, especially in this Unit – the attitude that they are children. It's very hard to break away from that. Yes, you've got to go through developmental stages to progress, but that doesn't imply that you need to use childish media, or childish teaching. You can adapt each thing you're doing into adult form. In music, we remember that we are dealing with adults. We never make them do what we wouldn't do. I can't logically put my finger on why it's wrong (some people will say, 'what's *wrong* with treating them as children?') There are people here who started off treating Special Needers as children – who have been shocked when they respond as a child never would. Something so antisocial, which a young child would never do.

So you might say that music meets a two-way set of needs for Special Needers. We try to develop a group: foster rhythm, encourage listening, and produce playing. And above all music fosters a conception of humanity. In return, I can get rewards from playing music and helping people develop their humanity.

## 4.00 Afterword

Not all day centres make it their business to deal with 'difficult' users with special needs such as the multiply handicapped. Most centres would exclude users who were aggressive or disruptive (like Godfrey) or incontinent (like Leanne). Some would not accept a user (like Rita) who was immobile and unable to walk. As Monday's users leave the Centre to return to their homes on the coach, it is evident that even the most vulnerable of mentally handicapped people, those with multiple handicaps, those who depend entirely on staff to define their social, physical and emotional needs, can be integrated into a larger group. No-one in this group will ever leave the day centre to take up a job, to set up a home or to get married. But progress needs to be measured by quite different criteria, such as whether Tom ever learns to place his cup *on* the table and his paint brush *in* the cupboard; whether Leanne can ever take herself for one whole day to the toilet.

Today's heavy needs and minute degrees of progress represent only a small group of mentally handicapped people. Leanne and her friends show that it is possible to develop interesting activities, to develop particular skills of movement and comprehension that stimulate and broaden everyday experience, that encourage sociability, that, in short, develop personhood.

Further, for the helpers, such activities can be of interest and generate enthusiasm. Monday has been a day of surprises. Here were some profoundly handicapped people, who nevertheless seemed as different from each other as chalk from cheese. We'd talked, eaten, spent an hour in a toilet, jogged, played lions and lion tamers, danced and played drums and tambourines. Today had been fun. Enjoyment was one expectation of staff in this Centre.

For it was not the routine which counted, it is what the routine meant to staff and to user. A session in the loo for Rita was not just a means of disciplining a lazy sphincter: Philippa saw it as giving relief to relatives, helping Rita's muscle physiotherapy, assisting her to gradually become more independent – above all, promoting greater human dignity for Rita.

# Tuesday

## Who's Who on Tuesday

*Clive* is Tuesday's man. Aged 31 years, he was born with Down's syndrome and has spent much of his adult life in day centres. He lives with his mother, now aged 75, who is a shadowy figure at the Centre. A natty dresser with a smooth manner, Clive has a mercurial personality which ebbs and flows from ebullient good humour to dark gloom.

*Olive* is Clive's care worker. She also heads up the Social Education department of the Centre and, in addition, is the deputy to Christine, the manager. A lively redheaded woman in her fifties, Olive is interested in the arts – particularly drama and music – and has a strong concern for social justice. She is married with children.

*Pat, Doreen, Len, Babs, Cath and Michael* are all members of Tuesday's Education group, which concentrates on self-care and cooking.

*Fran* a teacher. Trained to teach in the 'normal' school system, she is now adapting her skills to young mentally handicapped adults. She is quiet and hardworking. Outside the Centre, she is the mother of young children.

*Michael* is a member of the Special Education group, an extroverted and a persistent hand-shaker. His consuming interest at present is cricket.

*Pam* an instructor at the Centre, is gentle and tall. She leads the Centre's outdoor activities in sport and gardening. Her empathic understanding of the user's feelings originates from her own past experiences of being a client of psychiatric services.

*Margaret* visits the Centre weekly as a speech therapist, seconded by the local health authority.

Tuesday is another heavy summer's morning with leaden humidity. At 8.30 a.m. through the spy-hole window in the Italian cafe across the street from the underground station, the working world can be seen to emerge. Familiar faces – Philippa, then Jo – can be recognized in the scurrying crowd. The short walk from station to Centre leaves the noisy main road where lorries thunder to the north, and passes through a pleasant park (the site of yesterday's jogging), faced by newly painted Georgian houses with shiny french windows.

In the courtyard of the Centre, the coach spills its morning cargo. Philippa, today's escort, dismisses Clive. He is Tuesday's man. He shakes my hand graciously, with a formal courtesy, he is stocky and dark-haired, with a solemn expression, lightened by a frank smile.

Once inside the Centre doorway, Clive leads me to the library. He settles back into an armchair, legs crossed, manner alert. Conversation, however, is unexpectedly slow. I had expected, from the poise conveyed by his posture, that Clive would be a conversationalist. Instead we communicate like two verbally inhibited participants in a Pinter play. The following tape-recorded transcript of our encounter indicates that in the end we not only reached a kind of understanding, but Clive imparted information about his past work, his present activities, his future aspirations, and his sadnesses and joys.

9.00 Meeting Clive

| | |
|---|---|
| J.C. | I'm talking to people about what they do at the Centre, what they like and dislike. What things do you do here? |
| Clive | I do print. |
| J.C. | Print? |
| Clive | Drawing. Pottery with Digger. |
| J.C. | Pottery with Digger. |

Clive   I'll have a think. Lots of things.
J.C.    Mmm, what other things?
Clive   Lots of things.
J.C.    Lots of things. I know you do swimming, don't you?
Clive   Yes.
J.C.    So, what do you like best about coming to the Centre?
Clive   I like it.
J.C.    Do you? What do you like the best thing of all?
Clive   Pottery.
J.C.    Pottery?
Clive   And print.
J.C.    Pottery and print. What do you like about pottery? – What's the best thing about pottery?
Clive   Not hard work.
J.C.    It's not hard work?
Clive   Yes. No.
J.C.    Would you like to do *harder* work than you do at the Centre?
Clive   Yes.
J.C.    What would you do?
Clive   I worked out there once. [Points outside]
J.C.    In the garden?
Clive   No, at Pollards.
J.C.    In that factory over there? [A factory down the road]
Clive   Yes
J.C.    Every day?
Clive   Every day.
J.C.    For how long?
Clive   Start in the morning, have a tea break, then a lunch break.
J.C.    I see, but you don't go there now?
Clive   No.
J.C.    Why is that?
Clive   They sacked me.
J.C.    Oh, I see.
Clive   *Like that.*
J.C.    Why was that?

Clive   [emphatically] They sacked me.

J.C.   Oh, dear. So now, how long have you been coming to the Centre?

Clive   Oh, a long time.

J.C.   Have you? Two years, three years?

Clive   Two or three years.

J.C.   What's coming to the Centre done for you?

Clive   All right, lots of things.

J.C.   What things? Can you tell me more.

Clive   It's done a lot. Football. Football, yes. I like that.

J.C.   Has it made you get better at things?

Clive   Yes.

J.C.   How has the Centre helped you?

Clive   Oh, lots of things. Money

J.C.   Money, yes.

Clive   I'm happy more.

J.C.   Happy? Why is that?

Clive   I don't know.

J.C.   What about the other people at the Centre? have you got friends here?

Clive   Yes. Lots of friends.

J.C.   Who are your friends?

Clive   Oh, Alan. He talks funny a bit, you know?

J.C.   He does talk funny a bit, in his throat, yes. Anybody else who's a friend?

Clive   I've got a girlfriend.

J.C.   Oh? What's her name?

Clive   I've got a girlfriend now.

J.C.   Who's your girlfriend?

Clive   Margaret. She's gone.

J.C.   Margaret, yes. So the Centre's helped you by giving you money, it's made you happier and it's helped you by giving you friends. Anything else the Centre's done to help you?

Clive   I go out Tuesday to swim. Pam.

J.C.   Swimming with Pam, yes. I hear you are a good swimmer. So is there anything else the Centre has done to help you?

Clive   Not much
J.C.    Not much. Have you got any complaints about the Centre?
Clive   Yes.
J.C.    What things don't you like about the Centre?
Clive   More money.
J.C.    You want more money. Do you feel you don't get enough money?
Clive   No.
J.C.    Why not? Why don't they give you more money?
Clive   [changing subject] It's taught me a lot of things.
J.C.    Clive, if you could, would you leave, or would you like to still keep on coming here?
Clive   What you say?
J.C.    You'd like to leave or still keep on coming here?
Clive   No.
J.C.    You'd like to leave? What would you like to do instead?
Clive   I'd like to go back next door, work. [He uncrosses his legs, sits up and looks towards the door. He looks bored.]

Clive has indicated that this discussion has finished. He has noticed the others heading for the Social Education wing of the Centre and he is by now half-way out of his chair following them.

The difficulty about talking to Clive is not that it is impossible, but that it is time-consuming and requires a degree of inventive trial and error to carry the conversation along. By altering a phrase, or a word, and offering choices and options it was almost always possible for Clive to understand me. Clive's comprehension of language appeared to be rather more advanced than his own expression, but his concentration flagged rather faster than that of his interviewer. What was the Centre doing, then, about Clive's language expression and his concentration?

## 9.15 Care Group

Olive is Clive's care worker, the person in charge of the Social Education (or Social Training) Programme and the Deputy Manager of the Centre. She has a warm personality and an expressive manner. Older than most of the staff, she has worked with mentally handicapped people for some twenty years and she describes herself as 'long in the tooth'.

*Olive*   Clive is one of our most pleasant young men. You'll have noticed that he has great difficulty in expressing himself. One priority in his programme is to develop his speech. Despite the fact that he can look after his personal care – he can toilet and feed and wash himself – he is rather limited by his background. He lives with his elderly mother, a nice woman. But she restricts his life enormously. She won't let him go out on his own, or even travel alone on public transport. Now this is his biggest drawback and it makes it difficult for us to help him achieve the degree of independence of which he would be capable. It's an example of the way handicap is reinforced by social circumstances and family attitudes which are, in the end, more 'fixed' than the handicap itself.

   Today, you'll be able to see us doing our best with Clive. This morning he'll join my Social Education class for cookery first thing and then, after the break, he'll be part of the literacy group run by Fran, our teacher. After lunch, Clive joins Pam's swimming class (swimming is his forte – he's very good at it) and then later on in the day he spends some time with our Visiting Speech Therapist, who's here once a week. You'll find his programme outlined here. You might be interested to read his most recent summary report in his record file here, as this gives a rough account of where he's at.

**Clive's Programme**

| Today is *Tuesday* | *Wednesday* | *Thursday* | *Friday* | *Monday* |
|---|---|---|---|---|
| **AM 1** Social education (cooking) | Sports Centre (includes travel training) | Pottery | Social education | Social education (holding group) |
| **2** Social education (literacy/ numeracy) | | | | |
| **PM 1** Swimming | Free time (choice is education) | Pottery | Free time (choice is pottery) | Social education (library) |
| **2** Speech therapy | | | | |

## Summary Report on Clive

*Condition:* Down's syndrome, diagnosed at one year.
*Family:* Lives with his mother, a pensioner aged 75. Sister lives in London and is caring and interested – takes him out.
*Physical disabilities:* Speech difficulty.
*Emotional development:* Happy and responsible, pleasant and polite. He can be a leader (has acted as foreman) – plays practical jokes!
*Social development:* Good, he mixes well.
*Appearance:* He looks smart. Can attend to dress and hygiene alone.
*Speech and vocabulary:* This is limited – he can understand most of what is said to him – answers in monosyllables. Has a speech difficulty.

*Physical co-ordination:* Good. He has good movement and co- ordination. He swims well.
*Personal care:* Can toilet himself day and night, feed and wash himself.
*Educational:* Can copy name and shapes. Can tell the time. Limited understanding of money. Cannot read or write.
*Recreation:* Likes swimming, football and pop music. Enjoys boxing (his enthusiasm for boxing led to an aggressive incident).
*Priorities:* (1) Travel training. (2) Speech therapy.
*Other:* See assessment for further details.

*Olive* Our set of admin. records include the weekly programme you've already seen, as well as the annual summary on each client. There's also, as the basis of the work, a very detailed assessment. Now you'll see from looking at the assessment that it is clear that there are contradictions in Clive's progress. For example in the field of self-care he can clean his teeth, but he can't wash his own back. He dresses himself adequately, but doesn't know when to change his clothes. He has quite acceptable table manners, but he can't get on a bus by himself. He can print his own name, but he doesn't know the alphabet. He can make a bed and clean a room very effectively, but he doesn't know how to handle gas and electricity switches.

So yes, there are contradictions in Clive's daily capacity – but there are in any adult human being! (After all, how many adult males aged 30 make beds or clean out dirty rooms?) Obviously, the question of ability relates to social values. A barrister, or a diplomat, may be as domestically incapable as a mentally handicapped man, but can demonstrate his *independence* by employing a housekeeper (or a wife) to make his bed for him. However, the mentally handicapped man is not in a position to do this. He cannot demonstrate his independence by *not* making a bed – for Clive, domestic incapacity represents dependence, not the reverse. So it is not only the act of bed-making which counts, it's the social meaning attached to the act, and for

Clive being domestically capable is a step towards independence.

## 9.30 Social Education

Olive leads a group into the Education wing of the Centre. This is a series of smallish rooms, two set up as modern kitchens, one as a laundry; each taking perhaps a dozen people in comfort. We enter a kitchen, officially to join a cooking session. But first, Olive explains the Centre's philosophy of self-help, while seven or eight people buzz around washing lettuce, cutting cucumber and opening tins. Clive is busy with a colander and a floppy lettuce.

*Olive*   The first part of social education is self-help in the sense of maintaining the body. Hygiene and self-care and nutrition. The point is what every *individual* needs. You start with what they *can* do and reinforce this, and build up their expertise. Then you explore need. Sometimes this is elementary, particularly when people can't comb or brush their hair, or even wash their hands properly. Right from the very beginnings, you see. Someone like Clive is taught how to bathe and shower and to shampoo hair. The hygiene side's quite important because he does physical exercise here. But as well as hygiene, memory training is important – soap, flannel *and* a towel.

Many people appear, like Clive, to be able, yet can't do elementary things. Some certainly can't cut their nails (that's quite difficult). But it's also important to see when they need cutting so that they can go to someone and say, 'Could you do my nails, they're terribly long – they're tearing my stockings', or something like that. The whole area of self-care is so enormous and important that we can only pick out crucial things. Its importance was realized only recently. Now, all these people in hospitals, if they had the simplest self-care teaching could do elementary things themselves – like the toilet, washing their hands and face and dressing. If it had been done years ago, the nursing staff could have concentrated on teaching the next stage, rather than these elementary things.

At this Centre, in the past, before the present management, this place was really a work centre. So you had people with competent work skills who couldn't even comb their hair, or shave! It's incredible just how many competent people – like Clive – can't wash their hands properly, or clean their nails. We try to tackle things as fun and get people to enjoy doing it and to take pride in it. But often, at home, mother says, 'I'll do it for you.' Alas!

Another aspect of self-care is food preparation and cooking. There's always some process that someone can be quite good at – the less able can help – just like washing the lettuce. Learning to look at things, to identify objects, to smell – going out to pick the mint for instance! Two cook their own lunch every day. This means they have to think what they're having, collect the money, go out and buy it, bring it back and prepare it and make it and serve it – the whole bit! It's something simple as far as cooking goes, like beefburger with tomatoes, or sausages and baked beans. But quite a lot of complicated thought goes into this, especially the time factor. If we could have more people doing that each day it would be excellent, because it's an all- round thing – timing, money, change, going out of the Centre alone to shop, choices of food. But it takes time to monitor and we're a bit short on space. But it might be best for the group to explain what they do and how they do it. Everybody, come and talk.

Clive and seven others join Olive around the laminate-topped table, leaving half-washed lettuces and tins of beans in the sink.

| | |
|---|---|
| J.C. | What kinds of things do you all do in Social Education on Tuesday morning? |
| Pat | Cooking. |
| Len | Shop. |
| Pat | Wash up. |
| Clive | Dry up. |
| Doreen | Put away. |

| | |
|---|---|
| Babs | Wash table. |
| Len | Wash lettuce. |
| Michael | Cook sausage. |
| Pat | Put stuff away. |
| Cath | Clean sink. |
| J.C. | Now, do you do some of those things at home as well, or just at the Centre? |
| Clive | Yes, do them at the Centre and at home. |
| Olive | What things do you do at home, Clive, that you learn here? |
| Clive | Bathe. Cooking. Wash your hair. |
| Olive | What cooking does your mum let you do at home? |
| Clive | Egg. Toast. |
| Olive | Clive, can you think of any other things we do in Social Education on Tuesdays? You just went out and did something there, didn't you? |
| Clive | Shopping |
| J.C. | So where have you been today, to do your shopping? To a big shop or a little shop? |
| Doreen | Little shop. |
| J.C. | And what did you buy? |
| Michael | Ajax. Hovis. |
| Pat | Ryvita. |
| J.C. | And how much did it cost? Can you remember? |
| Len | Sixty-one. |
| Olive | Sixty-one was the change! |

10.30 Break

Olive and I leave the coffee queue in the hall and find a quiet room, so that we can talk at greater length about the Social Education department.

*Olive* Mentally handicapped people *are* slow learners. When they come here, they've only just started to cope with the essentials of life; learning is just beginning. We inherit people here who didn't previously have that chance, who left school and were put in a workshop and who were cut off at the time they should have been learning. So we have that backlog.

I can think of two people here who could read when they left school. Then they went into workshops where they did routine work-tasks. And without the reinforcement, and the principle of over-learning, they forgot their reading and writing. Nobody talked about signing on for social security, for instance, so they forgot to write their name. It was the recognized thing for the parents to get the social security. Whereas now, on principle, we like our people, if they can write, to get to the post office, to sign for their own money, to feel independent. Just a very small matter, but a fact that we had to deal with. Reading enough to sign on and to cope with notices is important for people's egos. When they go out of the post office they can see 'EXIT'. They can go into a shop and see where to 'PAY'. Very simple things, but unless they're taken out and about, with the idea of learning, they tend not to be motivated.

Training then, is to make them feel confident so that they can be more – if not completely – independent. In most centres, this never crosses their mind because they're always told what to do. The decisions are made for them and for a large part they're sitting (unless they're the hyperactive type) because it's easier for staff to deal with people when they're sitting. People can actually *deteriorate* in a day centre.

Some families encourage independence usually only to a lesser degree. Their feeling is that they're family responsibility, for life. Thus the fear of them making mistakes is pitted against encouraging independence. Of course, all young people make mistakes, but some parents just can't bear to think that *their* young person might go out and buy something that won't suit them. True, some parents train their children to clean their teeth properly, to bathe properly, to brush their hair, but very very few. On the whole, it is much easier and quicker for the parent to clean them – forever a child. When parents come up against problems, many tend to give up, whereas here it's not like that. We never give up and we try different ways. Whereas the parent would possibly say, 'Well, that's just not possible.'

It *is* difficult, if the parent and the centre don't see eye to eye on how far a person can go. Take Clive, for example. He was getting on very well, going out with a group and travelling on the bus. We would like to make him independent in travel, but his mother has told us on no account are we to let Clive out of the Centre alone. So that's a great handicap to developing more independence.

Another thing about mentally handicapped people is that they often have a very irregular pattern of achievement. Take Clive, he's very capable in many ways. He dresses himself and showers, yet he can't wash his hair properly yet. Someone who is not too bad at literacy, who can read well, may have very little comprehension. Other people have a great memory for dates, for people's birthdays, yet at the same time, they can't read. (If people look as though they're not going to be able to read, we try and teach them essential *words*: by repetition, copying, games, all kinds of methods, all the pre-reading skills have to be used to develop a 'sight' vocabulary.)

And then there's the group thing. We work in this department to get people to relate to others, because they are very lonely people. They are isolated. You've noticed if you come into the room that Clive always talks to *you* – he's not talking to his friends, but he has improved considerably lately. Generally, people here relate always to the member of staff, rather than to their peers.

I usually start each session with language, so that they talk and relate to each other. To discuss, not only their news, but to ask each other questions. (Something that they rarely do is to ask questions.) If they're telling you about an event, I get them to try to *sequence* it. To relate what they did to start with and to follow it through to the end of the day. It's very difficult, of course – some people do it very well, but the majority don't. Many people are quite disabled when you give them an item to sequence. But let's move to the teaching room and see how Fran, our teacher, plans a session.

## 11.00 Education

Clive, by now, is in the Education room where Fran, who teaches literacy and numeracy, has promised to explain her work. There are seven people in the room, all apparently working at different tasks, but Fran is with Clive, showing him pictures and asking names of objects. Fran suggests that I talk to Clive's neighbour, Michael, who knows the names, scores, batting and bowling averages of all the current England bowlers playing in the Test series against the Australians. His task is to write a story about his visit to the last test match at Lords. We discuss – completely in monosyllables – who should be England captain. Then Fran explains her job as teacher: what groups does she work with and what is she trying to do?

*Fran* I'm fairly new – early this year – so I'm still feeling my way. Overall, I do three sessions a week with the more able, which has been straight literacy and numeracy, with a bit of current affairs, and health education. Then I have another session with people who are withdrawn from other groups, and they're usually of quite low ability. I do 'very basic concepts' with them and they just come in perhaps for an hour, and then go back to their general groups. And I do a session a week with the Special Needs groups, again on 'basic concepts'. As time goes by you get a clear picture of everybody. I don't get anyone more than once a week, say forty altogether, an average of eight to ten a group. Bigger groups than we'd like, but we're short-staffed.

Oh, 'basic concepts' include things like putting across colour, and size and weight and that sort of thing. Then there's teaching the 'social sight' vocabulary; the common words people need to recognize, like 'BUS STOP', or EXIT'. It's more mechanical and is about learning one word at a time rather than learning language generally. Numeracy is difficult – you want them to learn about money and things to make them independent as adults – yet a lot haven't got the basic concepts of number. So you start at the beginning. Once you get into money it's quite abstract. If they don't really understand what 'one' and 'two' means first, it seems a bit of a waste of time.

With some that are older, when they were at school there wasn't a lot going on, or much reason to try and teach them things. With them, it's difficult to go back, but with the younger ones, you build on things which have already been done at school I'm never sure where the 'ceiling' is. In number and written work, the most able are all about six or seven years old. Of course, socially, there are things they understand that a six-or-seven-year-old wouldn't, or wouldn't be able to do.

One problem is motivation. There must be some kind of point to it for older people. I'd like to introduce more of a games element, particularly for number. That would be quite a good way of doing it for older people. More number games rather than just sitting down and doing sums. The same with literacy, you can do it around things like going to the cinema, or TV programmes, so you can link up number and reading and writing. Then there's more point to it – because if you want to go to the cinema, it's useful if you can find out in the paper what's on, and then read some of the signs on the way there and be able to handle your own money. This means you can always do more on your own, without always asking people.

Having the right materials is a problem. There *are* some books for handicapped people, but the ones I see are not very interesting. We hope to start making a few books. We could tape things that they talk about, things that they've been doing, and then put it all together in a little book.

Each person has a lesson format, developed from the priorities located at the annual assessment. Within that, I try to balance literacy and numeracy. At the same time I try and find areas of weakness, but I don't want to make it too mechanical. For example, some people are very bad on sounds, something I can follow up with phonic work. In number, I use the same criteria as a school, really. I've got a quick checklist of things – volume and length and weight, and so on. Some don't really understand number; a lot do it by rote. Even people who count quite well do it often by counting out. For a lot of them, there's no rhyme or reason to any of it, so I've been working with concrete materials all the time, trying to use as many objects as I can. Going on to money, which is obviously a priority for a lot of them, I know they do find it very difficult because they can't make that kind of jump, that this coin is worth a certain amount, and this one, although it's just a coin, is worth *two*, or *five*, or whatever pence.

Being a teacher *has* been a help. I have lots of different ways of approaching a problem and without teacher training I don't think I would have realized the importance of keeping it simple and using lots of materials. I don't see great academic leaps, but I do see improvements and I see people's self-confidence develop. And they're coping better, they are able to do more things than they could before and that's really good. Obviously some people are never going to go out and live on their own, but there's something they can do.

## 12.30 Lunch Break

From the park in the lunchtime sun, Clive can be seen in the distance, sitting alone on a fence outside the factory building next door to the Centre, posture slumped, face disconsolate. Clearly he has means of getting away from the Centre despite his mother's strictures. He looks unhappy, unlike the confident, poised young man of the morning. En route to the bank, I pass him sitting hunched on the wall. His sad face barely changes to acknowledge me.

'What's wrong, Clive?' I ask.

He grunts and points his head to the factory.

'Would you like to be back at the factory?' I ask him.

Clive grunts a reply and looks away.

Back in the Centre, I see Olive in the cloakroom and ask her about Clive and the factory.

'Oh', says Olive, 'that was a sad tale. About eighteen months ago, we encouraged the packing factory next door to take on two or three of our people for work experience. One of them was Clive. He went five days a week, all day, did simple jobs on the assembly line and absolutely adored it for about seven months. And then the work finished and they couldn't pay him any more. We were in a difficult situation. Should we continue to let Clive go to work, unpaid and thus exploited, or should we ask him to come back to the Centre? We didn't feel we could agree to him staying on in the factory unpaid and he has come back to the Centre. But we're not always sure that we've done the right thing.'

## 1.30 Swimming

The swimming group goes to the pool of the comprehensive school next door. Ten of us troop off with Pam the instructor in charge, and Jo. Men and women change in separate spaces. Pam explains to Michael that he must not look over the top of the wall into the women's changing room. In the pool, Clive has again become the friendly clown. He is the most capable swimmer – with his strong body he has a firm crawl stroke. For the rest, it is, says Pam, a matter of increasing confidence in the water. At first, the staff work with individual 'swimmers' – helping them to float and to put heads under the water. This is a quiet and disciplined time. Then the tempo changes as we divide into two teams for a ball game and energetically throw the ball to team members across the pool. Laughing and squealing, we come out of the water, dry ourselves, dress and walk back to the Centre. Whilst we dress, Pam explains the philosophy behind the Centre's sports programme.

*Pam*   Well, with swimming, first there's the exercise. Then, you can introduce quite a lot of discipline. They have to contain themselves in any sort of sports and games activity.

We do set up certain boundaries and then you find that you can relax in those boundaries, so it's combined with fun. Today, I took Michael to the pool for the first time and geared the session mainly around him and I was quite pleased with the way it went for him. Normally, there wouldn't have been so much on games. We usually finish with a games session, but we start off teaching something. Various things – one, the danger of water, that you can't breathe under water. There's a couple that are very, very wobbly. You might have to start off just teaching them to wade in water, just to walk in water. A lot of work has gone into basic teaching. Like Aidan, with Down's syndrome. At one time he'd just go under – he had no fears and he'd just stay under the water. I even felt at one time that he might be getting some sort of 'high' from staying under there until he was near enough unconscious. The only way I could really overcome that was by saying very clearly, 'out'. He understood that.

There are one or two that I think could swim. But the one thing I'm always telling them is they lack courage. I can't give that to them, it's got to come from within themselves, yes? Co-ordination can be a problem too. I don't know whether you noticed that today: they can't see their legs raised behind them. What I've been trying to do is to teach them to go on their backs so that they can see their legs.

Clive is the only one, actually, who can really swim. Some of them are deceiving! I mean I take another guy on Thursday. He can swim until you take him out into the deeper water and then he comes unstuck, because he's been doing two or three strokes and then kicking off with his foot!

After, there's the hygiene side. They have a shower to get the chlorine out of their hair and they wash properly. I think it makes more sense when they're doing hygienic things for a purpose. We also take a group to the sports centre on the bus once a week, for football and netball. We join up with two other centres, select teams for five-a-side football, and five-a-side netball. We get a fast game going – and a slower game with far more input from staff. There are certain laws we must stick to and they must contain themselves. For example they learn that they can't bash somebody up because they're losing, or whatever!

Sports do channel a lot of unused human energy into the right direction (whether it be sexual frustration, or aggression, or whatever). There's that pent-up energy that needs to be released: I think that's my main theme. But you get a lot of bonuses coming in on top of that, emotionally. For a lot of them, their bodies are adult. So there's got to be release somewhere. And OK, if you're saying that you can't allow them to have sexual relationships, then you've got to have energy channelled somewhere, haven't you?

Sports are important, not just because of the benefits of a release of energy and because people need exercise, but also because they need a bit of fun in their lives as well. It shouldn't be a trial, coming to a centre. There's got to be some sort of fun in it as well. Yes, again it's not only the energy release, or the fun or the exercise, it's a good way of getting across how to behave acceptably in the streets. Jogging or travelling to sports gets them out and mixing with people, seeing life, seeing what's going on around them in the park, down by the market. We talk about what we've seen when we get back.

We have to use public transport as well as the streets. They've got to know how the public expect them to behave, although sometimes I find the public very intolerant. When we go to the sports centre and the public cafeteria to buy a drink, I like them to sort out their own money. It's *their* money, *their* choice of what they're going to buy. But you get sarcastic remarks from people like, 'Oh, just as well we haven't got a queue!', or whatever. I get angry, I wonder what *they* feel: it must be quite painful, actually, to hear those sort of comments. People can be very insensitive.

Bus drivers, when they're getting on and off the buses, are often not prepared to wait. But it's a good exercise for them to realize their own limitations. For example, if you can't manage the stairs, then you don't go upstairs on a bus, because the bus won't wait. But I do think buses could be a little more tolerant!

The other extreme, where it's embarrassing, is when people are very patronising. There's no in-between. On the whole I think the public are quite frightened and they really don't know how to approach our people. Perhaps if they just approached them as human beings, or the same way you would anybody else, they might learn something. I think the public has got an awful lot to learn.

I was a 'natural' at sports, from school, and from childhood it was something I used to be very keen on. Funnily enough, I think it was something I'd always dreamed about doing – a job where I was introducing sports, games, or whatever. I didn't come to this Centre with those sort of ideas, but when I'd worked here for a while I could contribute in that way. Whatever group you're taking, you've got to have an interest yourself, you've got to have enthusiasm, otherwise it doesn't come off, onto the clients..

## 3.30 Speech Therapy

By now Clive has gone to speech therapy. The speech therapist is seconded to the Centre by the local health authority. She explains that working with the mentally handicapped is not usually seen as a priority for a speech therapy practitioner (as it is not for any practitioner – whether medical, social work or occupational therapy). Margaret, the therapist, is conducting a language group, which seems to be largely about making a cup of coffee. Action follows and then Margaret explains further.

*Margaret* The major problem that these people have is almost always that their comprehension is way above their expressive speech, so they understand a lot more than they use. So we get people to use speech more, directing other people and asking questions.

For Clive, for example, his understanding is at a three-to four-year level. But the speech that he uses is maybe at a two, two-and-a-half-year level. So it's just really expanding him and others. I didn't want to run the group like some language groups are run; the use of little pictures and just people responding to pictures. Obviously you end up using some of that, but I wanted it to be much more, related to more everyday things.

Like when we went to make coffee before, I stood in the kitchen and said while they made coffee, 'What do we do next?' I just got them to talk. Of course you get problems; they don't understand the questions that you're putting to them, so you have to be careful to rephrase. There are a few more verbal ones, so that helps the ones who are less responsive.

I end up doing a lot of listening. You know: 'Which of these words has a particular sound at the end?' I really found, working on an intensive individual basis, that habit was so ingrained that you could do very little to change their articulation. Someone like Clive – he'd probably be greatly improved if he opened his mouth and spoke out a lot more, and he only does that through increasing his confidence. The speech therapist who sees him individually does a lot more work on articulation.

When I first came, I started seeing people individually, then talked to their care worker and other members of staff so they could back up the treatment. It didn't work out; it was too complicated to cover everyone. So we decided to work in a group. I'd have a group of eight all morning and another speech therapist (who had half a day here), was to see group members on an individual basis. The group method works better. You have a whole afternoon, not half an hour, and it's good for them to talk to their peers.

I give suggestions to staff on ways that activities could be carried on into other sessions in the Centre; but that's the least successful bit. The staff look at speech matters, but you can't 'account' for all the different speech activities that each person is doing. So more time to communicate would help staff tell *me* how they're going about including speech ideas in the programme.

But this Centre is really unique, the staff are such a nice bunch, so interested in their work. One of the things I stress is that staff should be very aware of what they're saying to clients. They might be saying very long sentences so that the clients were missing half of it. One problem with mentally handicapped people is auditory memory – they just can't retain things for very long. These great long sentences: if staff could break these down, that would help. Some staff (not here) get into talking in abstract concepts and the clients are just absolutely bewildered. I have asked staff to test out how much the clients in their group remember related to their length of sentences. They couldn't remember a lot that was going on.

## 4.00 Afterword

Who goes where, when and why indicates that some very complex daily, weekly and even yearly planning takes place behind the casual friendliness of this Centre. But already, by Tuesday, after a day in Special Needs and a day in Education, I am aware that this Centre ticks over very differently to most. First, all the users have an individually prepared programme to follow, and second, most of the work with users is done in small groups. This contrasts markedly with other day centres, few of which have individual timetables for their users to follow: timetables which have been drawn up after detailed assessments of users have taken place. More frequently users come to the centre and fit into whatever is going on at the time.

There are no rooms in this Centre containing mentally handicapped people tucked away, working away at industrial or contract work jobs. Usually day centres have rows of tables with people sorting screws, packing envelopes or labelling toy boxes with varying degrees of concentration. Most centres for the mentally handicapped have most people working for most of the week and most centres tied their users to contract work. Staff in this Centre do not wish to be thought of as 'minders'; they have particular aims for users and generally have mapped out a method for achieving the aim. Over tea in the library, Olive explains her views about the attributes needed by staff who work with mentally handicapped people.

*Olive*   Oh, first I think the education of life is crucial. Yet, that's perhaps not really quite correct, because a lot of people on the staff here are young. But they are very capable. Yet I do think, as you go on in life, that you learn about the 'normal'. You have children of your own, and get to know the 'norm', right? You know about so many different aspects of child development, and you learn psychology as the practical application of theory, with human beings. Then persistence and inventiveness, to know how to approach somebody who seems to be completely rigid and set in a certain aspect, to know how to try and find other ways – no one way is right. Other skills? I suppose patience and observation are crucial.

Training is important. It gives you a chance to step back and have a look at the whole scene of the mentally handicapped: the hospitals, the different types of centres, and the different facilities, and the different methods of approaching the problem. You meet other people who are working with mentally handicapped people, you learn from other people's approaches. I must say I found my training most gratifying. It gave confidence and you feel you've got some expertise.

I've always felt that mental handicap was a 'bottom of the barrel' service. Very few people, comparatively, involve themselves with working with mentally handicapped people. There are more now, in all kinds of agencies, and the public is slowly, very slowly moving. When I came into the work years and years ago, I thought 'Goodness! This is terrible that such very nice people are given such a raw deal.' That made me want to continue.

One must get some sort of satisfaction out of it, or one couldn't continue to give. Obviously you give a lot of yourself to it, but you must get a lot back. the *little* improvements and gains are important. You've got to have certain satisfaction from what you're doing, otherwise you can't go on in this type of work, there are so many stresses and strains. I suppose I've always felt it was fascinating, because there are so many changes in people.

People outside say, 'How *can* you do it? I couldn't possibly do it.' They can say 'Ahh', and help someone across the road, or onto the bus, they don't see them as *people*, with character and personality – and they all *are* such characters and personalities! I suppose I think it is basically useful, useful work. And everybody likes to feel they're useful, don't they?

There *is* one important factor in working, in the stresses and strains of a centre, where we obviously try to do too much, or push ourselves. It is important that we have empathy together as a staff and that we all have a similar rationale and philosophy towards the work. If it was not so, you really couldn't take it. If there's not harmony, the clients are the first to sense it. You can't achieve the same results, you get the divide and rule, and backbiting. This is one thing that people notice at our Centre, that there is an empathy between the staff – a caring situation. We all discuss things openly – and if we don't, it's because there wasn't time. We don't take offence if somebody hasn't done something that they should have, because we know that they have different pressures, and one can't always be perfect.

I've worked in a number of centres, and I have noticed cliques. You don't get the same enthusiasm in the staff for the work, unless you've got that feeling of closeness, together. I don't mean you live in each other's pockets, but you do care about the way other people work, and follow it through, and talk openly about people's problems and don't take offence when people criticize, or make suggestions.

The first centre I worked at, I was told that if you didn't like the way things were run, then just to leave – 'Don't start trying to alter the thing – just leave.' (What a wonderful start to a job – 'Just go'!) This manager said, 'We've had a lot of people here that haven't agreed and it's no good trying to change anything; just go, or leave it as it is.' Marvellous!? The good atmosphere is a factor which is very important in working in this Centre.

Olive departs to do her shopping – by 4.30 the Centre is empty. Very few day centres – let alone hospitals – run complex education programmes for users and less than half the users of day centres in England and Wales ever attend *any* type of education class. If education is included as part of a day centre programme, literacy and numeracy classes are the most frequent, followed by shopping, cooking and domestic training groups. Few classes exist on self-care and very rare are classes in drama and music, such as the ones conducted by Mitch and Anil yesterday.

A few users in a few centres benefit from games or sport, but indoor games, such as table tennis or snooker, are the most common. Contrary to Pam's approach, sport is viewed as 'time off' from work rather than as a specific form of social education.

A minority of centres have a visiting speech therapist, but the combination of group work reinforced by individual work is unusual. 'Treatment', as defined by most day centres, means handling and dispensing users' drugs, such as tranquillizers or anti-epileptic drugs.

The difference between Highbury Grove and many centres is the belief that 'education is everything and everything is education'. Activities not considered strictly as education such as speech therapy and swimming or even drama are 'milked' for their educative potential and integrated into the philosophy of the Centre. The transfer of information and the overlap of work boundaries mean that the focus for the staff is not maintaining the 'purity' of a particular knowledge base, or preventing skills from being shared. Rather, knowledge and skills are subject to the basic requirement that people like Clive be able to talk more clearly and more often.

But what of Clive? He has joined the coach and gone home to his aged mother. The day centre takes up only 35 hours per week of Clive's life. The question is whether the other 133 hours will be more influential in shaping Clive's progress or lack of it. This is a topic to be discussed later.

# Wednesday

## Who's Who on Wednesday

*Paul* is tall, dark and hulking. His initial, frightening air results from his habit of looming over smaller strangers in misplaced friendliness. The focus of Wednesday's activities, Paul (and his behaviour) is regarded as one of the Centre's headaches.

*John* teaches art and is in charge of the arts and crafts programme. In his thirties, he is friendly and casual. Wears jeans. Comes from a commercial art background.

*Tim* is a user, now mainly an art student. Bespectacled, earnest and introverted, Tim wears a helmet to prevent damage to his head when he has fits. Tim's condition is a mystery – but as he has become a successful art student, he has relaxed and become more sociable.

*Digger* is a pottery teacher seconded from the education authority. Experienced, gentle and understanding, he spends two days each week at the Centre.

*Barbara, Doreen and George* are members of Digger's pottery class.

*Spiro* is Greek and communicates in this language at home. In his mid-forties, he has recently taken to pottery and sits absorbed for hours at the pottery wheel.

*Bob*, a quietly spoken art teacher who teaches drawing and painting, is seconded by the education authority.

*Margaret* is a former staff member, who has just moved from the Centre to manage a hostel. She was responsible for the Centre's video project, which turned itself into a therapeutic group.

*Seona* is an arts administrator who directs SHAPE, an organization dedicated to bringing arts and crafts to handicapped and disadvantaged persons.

## 8.45 Arts and Crafts Day

The third major 'department' in the Centre is the Arts and Crafts Division. An early inspection of the entrance hall of the Centre, before the arrival of staff and users for the day, suggests a busy department. The entrance hall, a large lobby, is hung with objects: by either side of the front door, huge pottery urns are filled with summer plants. These indicate the successful completion of a group pottery project – and also a project merger with the gardening group! The walls of the entrance are hung with a series of original paintings and lithographs, several announcing awards for the artists. Against the wall is a table, with pottery pieces marked for sale at affordable prices – mugs, bowls, urns, plates. Where the pieces differ from those at most centres is in the functional quality of most of the work. I select two planters and a dish.

Very few day centres teach pottery or painting: in fact, it is rare to find day centres which teach arts and crafts skills systematically: rather, arts and crafts are more frequently (and at times cynically) used as 'fillers' – activities to be used in an ad hoc way to fill in time and keep users quiet. The range of crafts is usually limited (restricted to sewing, kitting and embroidery, with a bit of woodwork and toymaking), the equipment is often non-existent or at best primitive, and there is no specialist arts and crafts knowledge amongst the staff.

Highbury Grove Centre, however, takes its arts and crafts seriously. A full-time instructor, John, is joined by part-time specialist teaching staff, seconded from the local education authority for pottery, drawing, painting. Sewing and embroidery classes are conducted as options by instructors on the staff – Cathy, for one, takes embroidery as an option group in the 'free choice' available on Friday afternoons.

It is clear that arts and crafts *skills* are taught at Highbury Grove. The therapeutic content of crafts is recognized as an important spin-off, but pottery sessions are not seen primarily as a therapy, nor is painting considered solely as emotional outlet. Rather, it is thought to be important that mentally handicapped people have access to systematic teaching of crafts.

So today we will visit the craft room where John leads a drawing/print group, to see how success at crafts can breed other successes. Then Digger explains the pros and cons of teaching pottery to mentally handicapped people after a group of potters explain their progress. Over lunch, Bob, the painting instructor, discusses how he assesses ability in his group members. After lunch, the staff meet to plan some further arts and crafts activities. Whilst strictly speaking neither an art nor a craft teacher, Margaret, a former staff member, has reappeared today, so there's a chance to talk to her about her video group. The day concludes with a live performance of a well-known mime group.


## 9.00 Care Group

Today's group meets in the studio, which accommodates about a dozen people at easels and tables, with an equipment room off at one end. 'Hello, hello, hello, hello,' says a six-foot-tall solid frame, hanging over me like a giant bat. 'Hello,' I say, retreating, physically and psychologically. This is Paul, Wednesday's person. John, the instructor, rescues me, introduces us and explains to Paul that a discussion may be in order.

Paul, as the man of the day, is marginally less dependent on the Centre than either Leanne or Clive for practical services. Whereas Leanne is totally *physically* dependent for her care, Paul is more physically competent: he can – after a fashion – feed, toilet and dress himself. Clive's limited speech and his inability to travel impose social handicaps which require the staff to protect him from the world outside the Centre. Paul, however, spends five days a week in the

Centre, but he is mobile and street-wise – being self-confident alone outside the Centre. In fact his restless roaming of the streets of London poses a different problem.

Interviewing Paul is not a great success as he is very strong and wants to take the tape-recorder apart. He considers there is no good reason why he should sit and engage in concentrated discussion with a stranger. He buzzes around, investigating paint, pots and the pottery kiln. 'Hello, hello, hello,' he repeats into my face. By now I have learned that his initially menacing air is not very real: he has a friendly grin.

Paul, aged twenty-one, has been at the Centre for about five years – he came straight from school. His parents, with whom he lives, are Cypriot immigrants, now living amongst their compatriots in North London. Paul's father has a small tailoring business and his mother suffers from repeated bouts of mental ill health which require intermittent admissions to hospital. Paul is her second mentally handicapped child: an older brother who also lives at home is handicapped.

John, the care worker, greets with casual bonhomie. He promises to explain the Centre's approach to Paul. Meanwhile, John is preoccupied with getting his group (with a high proportion of tall, thick-set and mildly rumbustious males) together. I have already gathered from random comments that Paul, now seated at a table (although thrashing his legs underneath) is considered to be one of the Centre's *challenges*. John comes to enlighten me and we move out of earshot to an equipment room at the end of the studio.

*John*  Paul, here, is quite bright in fact. But he has big behaviour problems. He roams around the streets on his own and he's been banned from the local library for pinching a librarian's bottom. He stops people in the street all the time and asks them the time. As you can understand, people are quite scared of him.

But the problems at home were our greatest worry. Last year, when his mum came to the annual review, she was depressed and said she was unable to carry on. We went into what happened at home with our psychologist. It seems that each day at Paul's house had a strange ending, quite bizarre. Each day, he went home from the Centre, ate supper, then went to bed – in the same bed as his mum. This was apparently a hangover from childhood when a doctor had told the mum to stay with Paul when he went to bed, to calm him down.

After a few hours in bed, at about 9.00 p.m., Paul would then get up and go out and roam the local streets for an hour or two. When he got home he would go to bed again. His mother set the alarm and toileted him every hour throughout the night. But despite this Paul always ended up wet in the morning. This pattern had gone on for 13 years and, needless to say, Paul's mum was complaining that she was worn out. The dad worked very hard in his business to make money and had always refused to help the mother with the children. Paul's older brother, also mentally handicapped, was at home all day. He was expelled from another day centre in the area because he was so physically aggressive.

Well, we got a plan under way after the review. You can see its essence in the following summary.

### From Paul's Review

*Action*
It has been decided that:

1   The staff are to ignore his bad behaviour.
2   The staff are to ignore his irrelevant conversation.
3   The staff are to discourage activities in the Centre which isolate him from others and to encourage group activities.
4   Encourage his use of the telephone.
5   Suggest to mother no drinks after 7.30 at night.
6   Suggest to mother that Paul changes his own bed.
7   Suggest that mother moves out of Paul's room.
8   Mother to report to Centre on things at home in a month.
9   A further review is needed in three months.

*Key workers:* John; Dana (psychologist).

Well, the plan has been quite successful. He sleeps apart from his mum for the first time in his life. He's wet less often at night, although he's not completely dry. And he's better at the Centre: he's less demanding now and not as disruptive of sessions. We've concentrated on involving Paul with his own age group and discouraged his solo forays out of the Centre. So you'll see that his programme, for the present, is confined to the Centre, except for going out with the weekly 'outing' and travel group led by Cathy. The others in the group have taken it on themsleves to control Paul, to warn him not to embarrass them or to draw attention to them, out in the streets! Inside the Centre the priorities for Paul are encouraging proper hygiene and trying to get him to take part in adult conversation.

**Paul's Programme**

| Today is | | | | |
|---|---|---|---|---|
| *Wednesday* | *Thursday* | *Friday* | *Monday* | *Tuesday* |
| AM Craft (pottery) | Social education (cooking) | Craft (printing) | Social education (Olive's holding group) | Social education (movement) |
| PM (Video) | Social education (Cathy's outing and travel group) | Free choice (drama) | Social education (literacy/ numeracy) | Craft (printing) |

Paul's main activities: print, video, social training, dance, movement.

## 9.30 Craft

The care group, made rather short on time this morning by my demands on John for explanation, disappear to the nether regions of the Centre and for five minutes the corridors are crowded with individuals hurrying to assigned groups. No-one seems to lead or control these changeovers – yet everyone appears to know where to go, and the corridors soon empty. Back in the craft room John is settling his morning group. As it happens, there are several members of his care group present in the craft group – Paul, for one. This is a print group, although the group are at varying stages of production and John is visiting individual artists and commenting on their work. Once everybody, including Paul, is working quietly we retreat into the equipment room and John explains his aims.

*John*  Well, the aims in crafts are just the same as the aims within other parts of the Centre, in social education or whatever. What's different is that the aims are transferred into visual terms, so that the craft becomes the vehicle or method for the aim. Like lino cutting. If you break it down, it's not purely about making a print. The thing is that somebody like Paul needs to use his hands, to develop his fine motor skills. So you give him a lino cut to do – that's a very good vehicle.

Why don't I sit ten at a table, each with a screwdriver, and ask them to put screws into plugs? Yes, that *is* using fine motor skills, I suppose. But look! Ten people are not the same, yeah? It's got to be a method used on an individual basis, not a means of containment. No, it's not just a matter of giving people something to do. It's where a method is applicable to the aims we have for a person.

OK take Rita here and Timothy there, they are just totally different in the level of their handicap and the skills they can command. Like, Timothy is quite good at fine motor skills – he can write and hold a pencil. But Rita, whom you know, she *can* hold a pencil, but to no end. And she's very immobile. So fine motor skills are the thing with Rita and you build on that. And the same with Timothy: even though he's more able, his gross motor skills are very poor. Now Rita and Tim are two totally different people, with varying skills but there's a common denominator, right?

Take another couple of people, who are more or less all rounders and not *too* bad; yeah, like Paul here, and Mike. Now Paul's hyperactive and dashes about and does things very quickly. While Mike is so bloody slow, you've got to pep him up and all that stuff while you slow Paul down. So you've got to wear so many different hats all the time, like what's good for one isn't so good for the other and vice versa.

I find it's a lot to do with how you approach them, like I talk to a couple of the clients with lots of joking and laughing – saying, 'Oh, you idiot, what the hell are you doing?' – that's OK. But you couldn't do the same with a different client. They'd burst into tears or get aggressive. You've got to get to know people well. You take this group of eight people. This morning, I'll change my attitude for near enough every person in that group. I do it subconsciously almost. Initially, my own method of assessing people is to let them do anything they want while I just observe. Then I see what they like doing and take it from there.

These people here have very limited experience, but even *that* is to varying degrees and entails a hell of a lot of different things like their family history. Are their parents old? Do they go out with them, or do they go out alone? Where have they gained their experience from and what type of experience is it? I think that their lack of experience is their greatest handicap and it's a common denominator in the broad sense. But if you break it down per individual, you could say that it's different for each one.

The same principles in craft relate to what's going on everywhere else here. It's a matter of giving people a basic experience. Say in cooking. In the education section, it's obvious. One way of doing it is to give people different tastes. One week we do an Italian meal and the next a Chinese meal and we get some feedback on the difference in taste. Which for some people is important (Down's syndrome people seem to have trouble with taste). So the whole thing of providing experience runs throughout.

Now, in craft, you can use portraiture as a vehicle. It's not just drawing a picture of yourself or someone else but to get people to see how they are composed. You've got a head with two ears (hopefully!). There's a nose, mouth and two eyes in a certain order in that egg shape! Then there's a neck on a body with two arms and what have you – all of a certain size. Now, a lot of our people just don't realize this. Some even don't know they've got a back! This comes out in hygiene groups. They have a shower and most of them never dry their back. They've never had to, because their mother always does it anyway – so they just don't know they've got a back. So for a person like Tim to draw this [shows portrait] he had to look at his face in a mirror first and we talked about it, then he came up with this. He wasn't into looking and seeing and translating observation into a drawing.

Take Tim. In a year he's gone from being a very stubborn, unsociable young man who would only do something he knew he could succeed in – which wasn't very much. He could count a bit, read a few words, but other than that he wouldn't do anything at all. That is until we had an amazing breakthrough on his artwork. Then he took off and started doing things (in other areas) which he just wouldn't have done before.

One day he was doing a drawing. It was based on his obsession – he counts red buses and flicks them off on his finger every time he sees one. The only way I could get him to do *anything* here was to work through his obsessions. So I said, 'Draw a bus.' We went through what a bus looks like, what a bus travels on. He would do that, he would sit down and draw buses. So over a period of months I gradually introduced him into lino printing for this one picture – buses. We transcribed it from the drawing into a printed picture. It took a long time, but he found he could achieve all sorts of things. He's had artwork in the City of London Artshow. And now he's an amenable character, too. He'll do anything you ask him to do – as long as he can find a good enough reason for it. Fair enough!

## 10.30 Break

John and I desert the noisy dining hall and take our coffee back to the quiet arts and crafts room. John is a trained graphics artist, formerly working as a commercial artist in the record business. So why has he forsaken commerce to work with handicapped people?

*John*   I went to art school and did a vocational graphics course, then worked for a record company and part-time in a graphics studio. I had x number of hours left over during the week when I saw an ad. which gave me the hours and money that I needed. I applied, not knowing what 'mentally handicapped' was: I'd envisaged that I'd have to wear a white coat all day and push lots of wheelchairs. But it was totally different to what I'd imagined and I decided to work here full-time. I started, on my own, a small print shop, an area that wasn't being covered in the craft programme.

I decided to stay. Anyone who comes into this work does it out of personal gain. Not in a monetary sense, but for work satisfaction. You're into desolate land: you can put your own stamp on things because you're working on your own a lot of the time. Given things like staff shortages, you've got to be responsible to yourself as well as to others. It's a good opportunity to experiment and discover you can do things professionally, not consciously for yourself, but for other people, i.e. set up a print shop or whatever.

I see my job here as trying to equip people to reach a better standard of living socially, by promoting independence and helping them be more aware. In specifics, it comes down to the raw material, the person. This man or that woman *could* go for a job in the forseeable future, but that is rare. The Centre is more to enable people to get by.

Teaching someone to stay on the dole or draw their cheque, for some that's good enough, just getting by.

Life-styles were different in the record business; and you didn't have to pay for it – you got things free! Free lunches, free drinks, free entertainment, free clothes and what you could make on the side. Here you don't even get a free lunch hour to go to the bank! But I wouldn't go back.

There are frustrations. The worst is that we are in an unreal environment. A day centre where people come and go is not 'real'. You know for a fact, when people leave here on Friday, they've got that weekend at home. And on Monday, you, to some extent, start again. For quite a time, it's redoing the same thing, over and over again. Then something will click and with someone, you can move onto something else.

I'm sure we are very confusing for parents sometimes. We treat these people differently. We are all the time trying to be *less* restrictive and get them to try new things. Parents must feel that it's all difficult enough, so why make it more difficult by asking them to do independent things? Not all parents resent it – but there *are* cases where parents are just as dependent on the kid – and the kid's handicap – as the kid is on the parent.

The large sizes of groups are frustrating, even though we work on a ratio which is small compared to most centres. I've got 1:8, which makes it harder to be working individually. You don't feel so bad working at 1:5. You can still only work with one person, but you're only ignoring four others instead of seven.

For me personally, one other frustrating thing is that I have to wear so many hats. As well as the art teaching, there's the care worker bit as well. You've got to be a sort of social worker as well as a nurse, and supervise the actual physical care – washing, toileting too. You're also the liaison person for your group. I'm a person who can only do one thing at once – if I'm taking a group, the rest goes by the board! People have to keep reminding me to deal with other things. Still it's part of the job and if I was doing that one thing, I'd get bored out of my mind. You're not just an art teacher in this place. And you don't just work for a borough here, you feel you work for the mentally handi-capped.

## 11.00 Pottery

John introduces Digger, a potter, who teaches for the Inner London Education Authority. Now, by choice, he spends two days a week in the Centre. Some class members in the studio today are his more able recruits. There are two activities. One lot are working on a group project: making a series of planters and urns to put in the new garden. Embryonic potters roll and shape sausage strips of clay to build the urn. Looks of absorbed concentration on the faces of group members suggest that this is a rewarding task. At another bench, four more potters are making coffee mugs from slip moulds. Digger explains that this is the beginnings of a project to try to develop a commercial product for the Centre to be *managed* by more able users. We ask the group members to join us around the table. Everybody, except Spiro, totally absorbed on the wheel, come to talk about the pottery class.

| | |
|---|---|
| Paul | We make things. We make mugs. And cups, egg cups, bowls. |
| Barbara | We made that, there. [Points to large urn.] |
| J.C. | Did you do that together? |
| All | Yes, yes! |
| J.C. | So what are you doing this morning? |
| Doreen | We're gonna tip the bowls into the . . . graveyard there . . . |
| George | [a superior aside] She means the moulds. |
| Barbara | Yes, the moulds in the graveyards. |
| Digger | Doreen calls these moulds 'graveyards', because they've got numbers on them. Like gravestones. |
| Doreen | In graveyards. You see them in many places, don't you, because they put a number on if anybody |

dies, don't they? They put the numbers on the grave.

J.C.  So you're going to use the moulds for clay. What happens then?

Doreen  We put them in the bath, down here.

George  Upside down.

Paul  And we leave them there.

Barbara  All the clay's at the bottom.

Paul  We leave them there to dry until it's finished.

Digger  Well, not *quite* finished. What do you do after you've opened them up there?

George  Put them on the side, on the table, take the lid off, like that, so that's loose. Then it's finished. It's a mug.

J.C.  What do you like best about pottery?

Doreen  You can earn a living out of it.

J.C.  Some people do, but not everybody. What do you like Barbara?

Barbara  [earnestly] I do like, I like the teacher. The teacher, he always learn, learn people.

Doreen  He's good to everybody.

J.C.  What other things? Do you like squeezing the clay?

All  Yes. Yes!

Paul  And rolling it out.

Barbara  And making sausages.

George  But now we've got to get on to finish this.

Dismissed by the group, I talk to Digger, to enquire what he expected when he came to work in this Centre three years ago.

*Digger*  It's difficult to say what I expected. I'm clouded by what I know now. It *was* just another place which gave more hours to add to my wages! Having said that, I discovered that I enjoyed coming here. I'm amazed by the quality of the staff. I don't know whether staff bring quality to the job or vice versa but this job does bring out strong feelings of responsiblity. If I could just keep one of the four places I go to in the week, I'd keep this place, there's such a good working atmosphere. I've been to other centres without the same degree of enjoyment – it's the community feeling, if you like. I think that most people can bear going to work each day to jobs, not because of the work, but because of who they work with – it's the community feeling at work.

Of course, the results compared to my 'normal' classes are very, very minimal. I don't get the same rewards in that sense, because you can't push the students in the same way. They achieve so little, but one reward is that *whatever* you achieve is such a big step – it's from nothing to something. There are great variations in my groups; some are so dull that they can only achieve on a play basis. Now today, they are an able lot. They like to achieve things. Normal adults are in the business of achieving things all the time: they go from achieving something to achieving a bit more; the step isn't so obvious as it is with this group.

I talk a lot in my class to explain the process and what use the results will be. Otherwise I'm just working in a vacuum and nothing is related to anything. A lot of them call it work, but I regard it as play. But a lot of them come in here to be paid (they are paid, at the end of the week – a very small amount). I'm trying to get rid of that idea: work is something you have to sit down and do until lunchtime. No, we're doing it because it's for the Centre, or for ourselves. Yet they're very conscious, even the 'dullest', that they're not normal. They are aware of normality outside. And that normal people work. And that they come here and a Centre is not the same. That's something we haven't thought through completely, that the 'work' aspect of it is quite important to some of them.

I like group projects very much. I'm always trying (without success) to get people in my 'normal' classes to look at what the other people are making. It's the most difficult thing in the world. Normal adults are too limited by their preconceptions, by their ambitions, and all sorts of things. It can be dreadfully frustrating.

Here, there isn't the same kind of possessiveness about the product. I started off by working individually and now, I don't, because it's a question of time and numbers. If you can get two or three people, at least, working away fairly happily doing something like a garden urn which is constructive, it allows me more time for people who are struggling for one reason or another. There are all sorts of reasons why people come in and don't do things. Like they feel sleepy because they're on tablets – which you don't fight. Also, just the physical business of running a pottery, having materials and processes together at the right time, takes a lot of time.

But individual work also has a place. When I started making pots, the fact that I could say 'I made that' gave me a sense of identity. It expanded me and gave me a sense that I existed outside of myself. These people need a sense of something outside of themselves. Some relate to what they make, very strongly, very easily, very quickly – 'I made that' – and they can recognize it: Spiro, for instance, he's a natural. For some, it's more difficult. It's such a big jump to remember from week to week, perhaps, or to have any sense of connection with something which is something outside of their bodies. They're not possessive in the way that normal adults are. Not that they've got much to share – and to be generous you need possessions, don't you? Some are generous, but not with objects so much as with interest and encouragement.

You don't need highly technical teaching. But to be a good teacher, you've got to know your materials and in that sense you need *more* technique than you're going to ever use. That's important. I don't think you can just get anybody in who did a bit of clay at school, or something like that.

[*Interruption: a middle-aged man enters*]

Digger   Hello, Spiro.
Spiro    Hello, my pot broke.
Digger   Which one?

| Spiro | The big one. |
| Digger | Can you mend it? Okay, I'll come in a moment. Perhaps you'd better start clearing up – can you organize them? [aside] It's alright, I like to leave them to organize themselves. They can do it by themselves. Spiro, I can mend the pot, if you can't manage, I think I know what's happened to it. [Spiro departs] |

Now to go back to teaching skills, one uses more technical information than one's going to impart. They're not interested in technical information in here, but the type of teacher is more important, because although he may have a lot of information, or knowledge, or techniques, it's not his job to muddle or to bewilder the ignorant. Spiro is a 'natural', he gets engrossed with the process and his hands have a rapport with clay. But even though he's an intuitive potter, it's important for him to develop as much understanding as possible of the process.

## 12.30 Lunch

Whilst Digger goes to undertake a rescue operation for Spiro's broken pot, John and I find Paul and we eat beefburgers and carrots and swap pleasantries. Usually, Paul is not encouraged to sit and talk with staff, but today he is invited to talk to me about his programme. We are joined by Bob, another instructor for the education authority, who teaches drawing. I ask him whether he considers any of his class numbers have real ability.

*Bob* Oh yes. See Theresa sitting over there? She is very good, in that she does look at things and she draws to a system. She has quite a lot of style. Some of her flower drawings, for example: she's got colours and shapes perfectly! she may just make them a bit more perfect than they actually are. Now she's done rabbits. Perfectly drawn. Once she gets a grip of something, she's pretty good.

But Theresa apart, most people in this group need to be motivated. I teach another class in a day centre for the physically disabled, they're all mentally OK. For them, it's just the difficulty of mixing the colours, the mechanics of it. They don't really need much motivation – they know what they want to do. Sometimes they need a little help, but generally it's how they're going to go about doing it. This group all get something different out of it. It's quite a sociable class: they do talk to one another. I can't really see any *dramatic* improvement in observation. I've done a whole term with flowers and they do look at them now more than at first. Sometimes you can't detect progress in a week, or in two weeks, or even in a term, but it's probably going on.

A lot of people lack confidence. They gave up painting, they were probably told that they were no good at it. But most people, in my classes here, with a bit of practice do get very much better.

Paul bursts in on our conversation insistently: 'Hello! Hello! Hello! Shake hands!' I am talking to Bob at present, I explain, but then Paul and I will play table tennis. (Paul wins.)

## 1.30 Staff Meeting

On Wednesday afternoons, the staff of the Centre meet. Today's meeting will be short because there is to be an arts performance in the hall by the visiting theatre group at the end of the afternoon.

If the staff are at a staff meeting, the problem is, who stays with the users? There is no adequte 'solution' to this difficulty. The current strategy is to designate Wednesday afternoons 'free time'. All users go into the big hall. There is a televison, table tennis, games. But, left to their own devices, most people just sit alone. A minority make a racket; a few do some exploratory snogging. Meanwhile the dozen or so staff sit in a semi-circle in the lobby outside the hall, one eye and ear on the agenda, the other on the hall through the glass.

The meeting is chaired by Christine, the manager, who welcomes newcomers and distributes today's agenda for discussion:

1 The current staff shortage – what action?
2 Gift of tickets for a theatre evening – who goes?
3 Developing the Centre garden – who co-ordinates?
4 A new work project – soft sculpture or 'inflatables' – how much investment of effort?

The *staff shortage* is discussed first, rationally but with controlled passion. At present the staff are minus two colleagues. Most frustrating. John considers that the Administration have been dilatory in advertising the posts. The effects on the Centre's programme have been a worry. First, the staff have had to surrender their 'planning time', a half day each week devoted to planning new programmes, completing records, making contact with other services for users, and so on. This is a blow to the quality of work. Second, the groups for which two new staff members would have been responsible have been absorbed into the workloads of the rest of the staff. 'Holding groups', that is, groups to 'contain' large numbers of users in a section where little individual or group work can be pursued, have been developed. However, John points out that he dislikes the holding groups intensely, because it reduces his task to 'client-sitting' (the Centre's version of babysitting). So, how is it best to convey to the Administration disapproval of the impact of the staff shortage on the quality of work?

Next, a prospective trip to the theatre. SHAPE, an arts organization, has offered eight free tickets to a West End ballet for an evening next week. Which users and which staff will go? There is no shortage of staff volunteers. Choosing the users is more complicated, but eventually it is decided that the six selected candidates will be asked to stay back with John at the Centre after the working day, to prepare their own supper, and to travel to the theatre on public transport. Getting people home late at night? Christine volunteers to drive all users home to their own front doors afterwards.

Next, there's the *gardening project*. Anil raises the use of the as-yet-undeveloped garden. A number of groups are interested in its use: the pottery group makes garden pots; the Special Needs group sits out in the sun; the gardening groups are busily landscaping the bare ground. So there is a need for a committee to co-ordinate a grand garden development design.

Then, the new work project. Jim designs and makes soft sculpture which he calls 'inflatables', as part of a project for the Mental Health Foundation. A week-long experimental project starts in the Centre tomorrow and Pam, nominated as the staff member to work on the project, has already spent a day observing the project at another centre. She reports that the value of 'inflatables' is an open question, to be assessed as the week goes on. John suggests that the 'inflatables' project can take place in the main craft studio.

## 2.15 Groups

In the interregnum between the staff meeting and the arts performance, I meet Margaret, a former staff member who has returned to the Centre to watch the mime show later in the day. Margaret has worked closely with Paul in the past and, in discussing this, I decide to question her more closely about her group. Therapeutic or counselling groups are extremely uncommon for mentally handicapped people: what could this method offer for other centres? I ask Margaret to outline the process of the group.

*Margaret* Originally, it wasn't a therapeutic group. Two years ago, video was brought in to try to suggest more positive ways of interacting, to try to teach some down-to-earth social skills. The eight members were all people who got a lot of negative responses from others, like Paul – because of the ways that they abused others physically, or verbally. We'd try using video so that they'd role play, and see themselves in different moods.

In the beginning we did anything to bring awareness of what they were saying to each other. A lot of work, right at the beginning, was about posture. Posture showed you what kind of a mood somebody was in: anger, fear, unhappiness, or lack of confidence. They started, after a few sessions, to pick up on how people were looking – sad, excited, or whatever. Role plays didn't work very well: they were more playing with objects around them rather than getting into a role. At that stage, it was too much of a leap. Then we used the empty chair technique, that gestalt idea, where you talk to someone who isn't there. What I said was: 'If there's something you feel you'd like to say to somebody, but you feel you can't for whatever reason, because it's not acceptable or because you're too frightened, or whatever – try saying it to that empty chair'.

I really didn't think it would work, so I was stunned by the response. Well, I think three people nearly killed off their mothers! They shouted at the chair, knocked it over, hammered it, and said a lot of things which presumably parents say to them. Like '*Be quiet!*' Or they'd knock the chair over: 'I shan't let you get up until you do as you're told and promise to do as I say all the time.'

One day, the video was stolen from the Centre. We became a talking group, rather than an acting group, free to talk about whatever they wanted. This went through stages. There were three main themes and it would depend very much on what had been happening in the Centre as to which they used. But the basic themes were death, sex and birth.

*Death* would come up at special times. When the group changed, after it had been going for nine months, it was felt that three people weren't getting anything from the group. Two went into another group, and another – the youngest – went off and did craft. She'd been the baby of the group, although I didn't think she was getting that much from it. But the group felt her loss really strongly and that brought on the first discussion that they'd ever had about mental handicap. This was quite freaky at the time to me, because I hadn't been used to hearing them talk about their own handicap and hearing how they felt. And they were saying things like, 'It's *terrible*, the way people stare at you in the street' and, 'Why do people do that?' They were asking about who *was* handicapped in the Centre and who *looked* mentally handicapped. Were the staff mentally handicapped too? They wished they were 'ordinary' (not a word I would use). They thought that ordinary people ridiculed them and laughed at them, so that was the link.

They asked me how I'd feel if I had a mentally handicapped kid. A couple of them said, 'I know, you'd send it off to boarding school'; and then somebody said, 'No, you'd just throw it in the bin.' It was incredible, this feeling of rejection. And in the group sense (which I wasn't really grasping at that stage) it did seem to have been brought on by the fact that I'd thrown out the baby of the group.

*Sex* was used to push the limits of the group and to see what I would tolerate. They could get obscene and I'd never stop them (which they found very threatening). This was more to do with the group dynamics than the subject, because they would just push and push and push. *I* felt quite threatened by it. (Especially the threat of somebody else walking into the room and hearing it!)

*Birth* was usually an expression that they would like to have their own children, or it was talking about why *I* didn't have children (some of which used to make me feel uncomfortable). Some of it was, I think, a desire to have somebody *themselves* to look after, because they were always being looked after by others.

After the 'baby' went off, that left a hole, because there was nobody for the group to look after. The death theme took a long time to come out. We had weeks and weeks of sessions where we had people walking out, slamming back in again, and bursting into tears. Death only had to be mentioned, or it didn't even have to be mentioned, somebody had only to think it was mentioned. (They were actually assuming that somebody was saying something completely different.) Also three of the people in the group had actually had a recent bereavement, had lost one parent.

But the main thing was an ambivalent feeling towards their parents, in their wishing that they were dead. One member threatened suicide (in the last few weeks of the group when they knew I was leaving the group and the Centre). It's quite common to say, 'look, I can't cope,' I didn't believe it would happen, but it threw the rest of the group out. This brought how they saw death into focus. (Before that, death was something everybody got upset about, talk about people they'd loved who died. They always linked that with people going away; staff, or friends who'd left here.)

Their understanding of death wasn't the same as mine. Either they talked about death as if the body was dead, and the thought processes were just trapped inside the head. Or the feeling that death was just going 'up there' to heaven, not much different to life except that you'd leave a few people behind, but you'd meet a few others that have gone. A Christian view of death.

They kept things confidential to the group. For example, there was one incident on the day that we'd been 'talking' to empty chairs. Afterwards, a few of them (including Paul) went into the dining room and started throwing chairs around. A member of staff really told them off and that made me sit up and think – we had to talk about what the group meant. After that, they were very protective of the group, and didn't like intrustions. If anyone came into the room, they'd say 'hurry up' and sort of 'get out'. And one said that she'd told a friend something that had happened in the group, at her break time, and they came down on her like a ton of bricks, and said, 'It's nothing to do with her. She's not in this group. You don't do that.' So they got very worried about confidentiality.

There were changes, in people. But of course it's very difficult to tell if the changes were to do with the group alone or with other things happening in the Centre. Paul, who *always* got negative attention, who always pestered staff and was really difficult – he changed. He was upset by the group, very early on. To start, we did eye contact and handshaking exercises. We'd just say 'hello' to each other and look each other in the eye. That reduced him to tears. After that, as soon as he walked into the room he'd be terribly upset. But at the same time, when he'd done it, it was something really precious to him that he'd managed it. I definitely saw – all the staff saw – an improvement. Obviously he relapses! Clive didn't really participate – he sat and listened. There were times when we talked about mental handicap and he didn't want them to talk about that. He looked pained. I asked him if he'd rather go out until we'd finished, but he stayed – I don't know whether it had any effect on him, but he certainly always came and sat it out. The only things he really joined it on was the obscenity: he enjoyed swearing!

I worked with our psychologist at the beginning. Then she was off sick for a few months, when things seemed to get very heavy. I knew there was something happening and wasn't sure whether I should carry on, whether it was dangerous emotionally. I had bad worries and asked if I could have supervision. Norman, the head of another centre and a group analyst agreed. Certain qualities are very important in leading groups and it made me look at what I was doing, in detail.

## 3.00 Performance

John announces the start of today's threatre performance. Paul sits in a middle row, actually still! A leading mime group, THE MOVING PICTURE MIME SHOW, is here. Whilst they are setting up a stage and dressing room in the dining hall, now to become a theatre, an expectant audience seats itself. Friday's sponsor of the performance is the artistic group SHAPE, founded as an arts organization to take community arts to the disabled and deprived. It organizes performances in hospitals, prisons, old people's homes and day centres. It takes thousands of physically disabled and mentally handicapped people to theatres and sets up workshops, seminars and groups. (For example, Mitch's Monday drama group started life as a SHAPE workshop. This was so successful that the Centre co-opted Mitch and the drama group into its permanent programme.

SHAPE uses Highbury Centre to 'float' artistic balloons. Today the MOVING PICTURE MIME SHOW are performing for mentally handicapped people for the first time and the purpose is to assess this performance for a tour of such groups. Their first piece is about a group of students taking an exam, supervised by a strict teacher. An introduction by an American mime artist explains that the performance is about 'the professor at the end of the semester marking grades'. The mime is lengthy and received with increasing restiveness by Paul and others. An unlikely piece to present to a group of people who are, by definition, academic failures?

The next mime is better received. Two men keep fixing a motor bike which keeps stalling and breaking down. This appeals to some male members of the audience, particularly Paul, who laughs uproariously. Are the actors aware that Paul, and many mentally handicapped young men, yearn for a motor bike: the zenith of macho ambition is to ride a motor bike of one's own? Perhaps achieving this vicariously in a mime show is better than nothing for Paul? None of us really know.

*Seona Reid* (Director of SHAPE) SHAPE links two kinds of people: on the one hand, those who are cut off from access to creative and artistic activities – the disabled, the old, ill, handicapped, the homeless. On the other hand, there are musicians, painters, dancers and other artists who enjoy working with and for such people. SHAPE simply brings these two groups together.

It offers the mentally handicapped opportunities for personal and social development. The experience of enjoyment and creation helps to build greater self-confidence and independence in handicapped people. It enables the artists to develop professionally and at the same time make a valuable contribution to the community. So SHAPE is a catalyst.

## 4.00 Afterword

Paul shakes hands with ceremony. He has enjoyed the special attention of the day. He lopes off into the street. Today has been an introduction to growth and pain, the existence of which tests the inadequate view that a mentally handicapped person is the sum of his or her IQ rating, or a test score. The actuality is, as John has pointed out, infinitely more complex and challenging.

Margaret's group made it clear that many mentally handicapped people have very strong feelings about how it feels to be classified as 'stupid' and are aware that they are 'different'. Whether or not they label themselves with an official diagnosis ('I'm a Down's syndrome'), many are aware that they have a problem. 'I'm very slow at doing things. People get cross with me, but here [at the Centre] they understand and know I do my best.'

David, in his early twenties, described himself as 'handicapped and backward'. 'I've always been like that, I couldn't get on with reading and arithmetic at school. People should be more understanding. People try to take the mickey out of me. It disturbs me and makes me feel nervous.' While some mentally handicapped people feel they have a disability of some sort, others think they suffer from a vague sort of mental disorder. 'Nerves' were seen as the most common cause of the condition. For instance, Christopher said, 'I'm a bundle of nerves.' Or birth injuries are sometimes viewed as the cause of their problems. 'It was brain damage when I were born that caused it.' 'I had an accident at my birth.' 'It was a bang on my head when I was born.'

Sometimes, the mentally handicapped person seeks explanations for disablement beyond the limits of their own body and mind. 'I have magic beings in my head. They protect me from seeing or hearing things that I don't like,' explained Diana. 'I have a man who talks in my head and makes a lot of noise,' says Phillip. In these two cases, these fantasy guests appeared to be largely benign, but for Vashti, uninvited guests in the head were confusing and distressing – and the cause of endless arguments about medical diagnosis between doctors in mental hospitals and subnormality hospitals.

Wednesday has confirmed that mentally handicapped people have a shrewd idea of what those who are 'ordinary' feel about them. They are aware that their neighbours look the other way, or cross the road to avoid them, or that people stare at them on the bus. 'People could help by understanding and helping you and not laughing at you,' says 16-year-old Simon, with Down's syndrome. 'I do like people to be friendly,' comments Petula, a 17-year-old. 'My neighbours should get to know me and talk to me and be nice to me. They should pay attention to me when I am ill and talk to you when you come out of the door.' 'My neighbours could be more friendly. They keep to themselves. I think they should say good morning,' muses Margaret, a 25-year-old.

So mentally handicapped people – even the apparently hardboiled, like Paul, know how it feels to be rejected and rebuffed. They are very sensitive to nuances of attitudes. This sensitivity has rarely been explored as a tool for creative work. It combines with an openness which expresses naturally feelings of sadness and joy. What can we do to foster a communal atmosphere, where mentally handicapped people feel 'safe' to share their anxiety and pain?

# Thursday

## Who's Who on Thursday

*Dee* is a sociable young woman who has made enough progress in the past year to lessen her dependence on the Centre – she has an unpaid volunteer job half a day a week in a day nursery. She likes her volunteer job and working in the kitchen at the Centre.

*Sheila* is a care worker and instructor. Originally trained as a social worker, she decided to work with mentally handicapped people and the day centre is her first job. Her main programme interests in the Centre are music, movement and drama classes. With long dark hair and an ethereal manner, she sometimes seems to be on a different plane.

*Sam, Ann, Clive, Rodney and Barbara* are fellow travellers on the bus to Ashley Road.

*Michael* is the Director of the Ashley Road Social Development Centre.

*Cathy* who takes a group on travel and outings, is also in charge of the Special Needs Group (see Monday).

*Clive, Mike, Doreen and Rodney* are some members of the travel and outings group. Rodney is also 'Shop' this week – he serves tea and snacks in the mid-afternoon.

*Olive* (See Tuesday) is Deputy Manager and a mother confessor.

*Tricia* is a student for the Certificate of Social Service (CSS) and is on placement at Highbury Grove Centre. Her paid job is in a hostel.

*Dee's mother* Mrs. Smith, is a mother who disapproves of the staff at Highbury Grove Centre, their activities and their aims for her daughter.

## 8.55 En Route

On Thursday morning at 8.55 a.m. Dee, with neatly cropped corn-coloured hair, an angular figure with a precise pattern on her blue shirt, gets off the red doubledecker bus and walks half a mile from the stop to the Centre. That Dee can catch the bus to the Centre is regarded as a minor miracle. But Dee's bus catching is due less to the inspiration of the miraculous than to the perspiration of hard work. For months, Dee has practised travelling on the local buses, remembering their numbers and their routes. Now, for the last month, she has been able to travel alone.

Dee is a friendly young woman aged 20 with a businesslike air. I noticed her on Tuesday in the background of the cookery class. When she is at work, particularly in the kitchen, deft confidence and calm authority take over from angular awkwardness. She iced a cake: cavalier sprays of icing across the top layer, flourishes of the spatula like a circus swordswoman. Then cherry and silver ball decorations lined up in workmanlike, if crooked, rows. But this Super-cook, of purposeful and brisk movement, of aesthetic gestures with knives and spatulas, could give way at any moment to a child, who stops and sucks loudly on the spatula, with blissful, unhygienic enjoyment. Super-cook and Suckling Child coexist in Dee.

This had been my introduction to Dee. Her weekly programme concentrates on activities in social education. In fact, until a fortnight ago, Dee had been away from the Centre for six months, attending a special course at a centre known colloquially as Ashley Road, more officially as the Social Development Centre, where tailor-made courses for members of the Centre attempt to accelerate learning in a particular area of deficiency or difficulty. As it happens, Dee is to revisit her tutors at Ashley Road later in the morning and I am invited to join the expedition.

From Monday to Wednesday, most time has been spent largely within the four walls of the Centre visiting the three major departments of Special Needs, Social Education and

Arts and Crafts. But Highbury Grove Centre tries to be a centre without walls. So today, most of the time will be spent visiting external activities. Of course, most day centre users spend more time out of the centre than in it – 35 hours or so at the Centre; the other 133 or so hours of the week users spend with their family, or the hostel staff. On this basis, Highbury Grove tries to recognize that a day centre should not be a 'closed' instutution; that a merger between the Centre and the rest of life is required. So today's time will reflect some of the things users do outside the Centre.

But first of all, Dee, and her care worker Sheila, explain what they will do today. Then Dee, five others and I will travel, by bus, to visit the Ashley Road Social Development Centre and I will accompany them to meet Michael, the Director. At lunchtime, back at Highbury Grove, Olive is to discuss the pros and cons of work placements outside the Centre. Then, in the afternoon, I shall visit the Travel and Outings Group who are, with Cathy, preparing for an expedition. I discuss some complaints about a hostel. At the end of the day Dee takes me home to meet her mum. Finally, there's to be a parents' meeting. All these things signify that as much, if not more, goes on outside the four walls of the day centre.

## 9.00 Care Group

Dee has found Sheila's care group, which meets in one of the Education rooms of the Centre. Sheila is engaged in a lengthy discussion with users about next year's summer camp: Dee and I move off to the kitchen to talk. Dee seems to enjoy a good talk; we discuss what she does, what she enjoys most and what she would like to do next. But first, we discuss how she gets to the Centre; how she has begun to travel alone.

Dee    Oh, I get the 143 to Highbury Corner. I get off and I walk down here on my own, and then I get the same bus going home. Sometimes, I get the same bus as

Mandy and we walk down together. If I meet her in the morning, she gets the same bus, we get off at the same stop and walk down. She lives in the hostel. I live a bit further along.

J.C.    And what do you like doing best here at the Centre?

Dee    Oh I like cooking, needlework, reading, writing – and a little bit of number work, not a lot. And exercising, with Sheila. And I do like doing travelling and outings.

J.C.    In all, do you like coming to the Centre?

Dee    Yes [uncertain].

J.C.    What's it done for you, do you think?

Dee    I used to do gardening, but I stopped it. I like doing needlework, silkwork. I do a lot of reading with Fran on Thursday afternoon – reading and writing. I like helping to dry up, and putting things away, so they're in order, and washing the tables – and sweeping up and that, and doing the things that I can do. I can peel potatoes, I can open a tin of beans, I was forgetting that. It's difficult to do the bread, but I can do eggs and other things now.

J.C.    What sort of things don't you like about this place?

Dee    I don't know really, I like everything, mostly. I like coming to the Centre instead of staying at home. I get a bit bored staying at home on my own. I have something to do.

J.C.    Dee, can you tell me about your work?

Dee    Yes, yes, the nursery?

J.C.    What do you do?

Dee    Look after babies, wipe tables down.

J.C.    What do you do with the babies?

Dee    I have to look after them.

J.C.    Look after them . . . ?

Dee    And put nappies on.

J.C.    Ah!

Dee    And then I go to get the shopping for the nursery, to get the coffee, milk, sugar and whatever.

| J.C. | What's that for? For lunch? Or tea? |
|---|---|
| Dee | No, for tea. I get the biscuits for them, for the mums. I would like to go all day but I can't. I have to do half time in the morning, then I come back here for dinner, like. |
| J.C. | How long have you been going to the nursery? |
| Dee | Oh, a long while, quite a long while. |
| J.C. | And do you get paid? |
| Dee | No, I don't get paid there – no. |
| J.C. | Dee, if you got a paid job, what would you like to do? |
| Dee | I would like to do typing and that. |
| J.C. | You wouldn't want to work with babies and children, then? |
| Dee | Yes, I would like to, one day. But I'd like to do typing on another day. |
| J.C. | Dee, who do you live with? |
| Dee | My mum, my brother and my uncle as well. My sister's married and has got two little boys. One's ten and the other one's four. I go down there now and again, they live in Wormsley, by the river. I did have a Nan, but she's not with us any more. |
| J.C. | What other things do you like doing, when you're not at the Centre? Do you go out sometimes? |
| Dee | Yes, I go out sometimes. I go away for the weekend. I have days off from the Centre and go shopping sometimes. And I get the right change. I help my mum in the garden. Would you like to come to see it? |
| J.C. | I'd love to. When do you think I could come? |
| Dee | I'll go and phone my mum now. You could come home with me today. |

Dee and I move off to the public phone box in the Centre foyer. Dee dials the number carefully, tells her mother that she has a visitor and then puts me on the line to explain. That done, I return to the care group base to look at Dee's daily programme.

## Dee's Programme

| Today is | | | | |
|---|---|---|---|---|
| *Thursday* | *Friday* | *Monday* | *Tuesday* | *Wednesday* |
| **AM** Cooking | Kitchencraft | Cooking | Work placement | Movement |
| **PM** Literacy/ numeracy | Needlework | Literacy/ numeracy | Literacy/ numeracy | Free (embroidery) |

Dee's programme confirms that she spends most time in the kitchen and the classroom. But because she only leaves the Centre once a week for volunteer work based on a council day nursery, this indicates that her dependence on the Centre, whilst modified by a volunteer post, is still substantial.

It being 9.40, Sheila has moved off to her movement class. She has suggested that I join her there to discuss Dee's programme before going to Ashley Road. In the hall, the sequence of activity goes something like this:

*Sheila* S-T-R-E-T-C-H and B-E-N-D, S-T-R-E-T-C-H and B-E-N-D. We pick up a *thimble* with our toes, we have our *trunks* like trees; as free as a breeze; and we whistle like the wind. We are visiting an orchard in the early morning, as the sun comes up. We S-T-R-E-T-C-H, on tip toe, to pick ripe peaches from trees, from under the nose of the farmer. We B-E-N-D, putting peaches in our baskets. We lie, outstretched under the trees, B-R-E-A-T-H-I-N-G in-out, in-out, smelling the fragrance of big gold-pink summer peaches.

[At a convenient moment, I interrupt Sheila's orchard in the Cotswolds and we sit on a scruffy mat in a London building to discuss Dee's progress.]

As you know, Dee's been away from us for six months at the Social Development Centre in Ashley Road. In that time, she's become much more independent, much less of a baby – she was a bit inclined to sit down and cry if things didn't go exactly her way before that. And above all, she learned to travel, alone on the bus.

The biggest thing for her now is her work placement at the nursery. She goes one morning a week to the pre-school nursery at the North London College, to try to develop experience in working with small children. We also felt she needed more of a sense of responsibility. But perhaps you could talk to the staff of the Ashley Road Social Development Centre about why we have made these recommendations?

## 9.50 Outward Bound

Dee and I make for the bus stop, to catch the bus to 'Ashley Road', in another part of the borough. At the bus stop we meet five young people from the Centre who are off to visit Ashley Road too: Sam, Ann, Clive, Rodney and Barbara.

Polite and unselfconscious greetings take place. The bus arrives, each pays the driver, and sits at the back of the bus, chatting quietly. They are a very well-behaved group of young people in jeans and T-shirts. Unspoken questions from fellow-passengers hang in the air. In this past week, newspaper stories and comments have concentrated on the right to surgery, and thus survival, of a new-born baby with Down's syndrome, rejected by parents. Arguments for and against continuing the baby's life spread from the High Court to suburban streets. The bus passengers have noticed the visible stigmata carried by some of my mentally handicapped friends – the classic features of Down's syndrome. They are carefully listening to our conversations. I am proud of my six young friends; glad that they are including me in their group. If the refusal to offer medical treatment to the mentally handicapped rests on their impoverished quality of life, this reduced quality is not

evident in these happy young people on this bright summer
morning.

My young friends sound the bell and escort me off the bus
towards a three-storey semi-detached house. This is the
Social Development Centre, known as Ashley Road. Dee,
as recent alumna, acts as hostess and shows us into the
living room. She finds photograph albums and memorabilia
of the last year's holiday trip to Ireland. Then she conducts
me around the garden, thick with courgettes, lettuces and
tomatoes. Inside, the lower floor of the house is furnished
like any home: lounge, dining room and kitchen. Upstairs
there are bedrooms and on the top floor, classrooms and
offices. At the top of the stairs Michael, the Director, invites
me to his office. He tells me for whom the Centre caters and
what he considers to be the priorities of the programme.

*Michael* For four years we've offered further education for
those between 18 and 25, at a time when mentally
handicapped young people leave school and go into places
with only limited facilities for education. A lecturer appointed by the education authority does the bulk of teaching in
literacy and numeracy; our students do go out to college but,
as well, the lecturer comes here, so that literacy and
numeracy is always reinforcing the practical work at the
Centre. (College courses – OK, they're good – but they're
classroom-based and bounded.) We have other specialists,
for example a craft teacher, a specialist in health and
hygiene and in sex education. The core staff are appointed
by social services, so we're a nice bridge between health,
social services and further education.

We take six to eight people at once and have a
staff-student ratio of 1:1. Mostly, our recruits come from the
two day centres in the area. To make it work, quite sensibly,
the more able *are* selected. There *is* a point at which certain
people can't come here, because they can't travel or are not
likely to travel independently. That's one frontier, one
overriding selection criterion. But we're heartened at who
can be taught how to travel alone. People *have* achieved

independent travel, and very quickly too. So much of what we do involves people travelling out, often without a member of staff. It negates the point to have people bussed in here. So that's where we start. 'Can someone already travel?', or 'Have they got the potential to travel?' And if so we'll try. We'll even meet them at home each day and bring them here for the start.

At the beginning some parents felt that Ashley Road was a kind of finishing school, a graduation machine, and their children would go from here into jobs. Now we say to parents: 'Look, there's no way that people are going to get a job at the end of it. Two people have, well that's wonderful, but a job is not an overriding aim.' Otherwise students and parents think they've failed if they haven't a job, when they've achieved all sorts of other useful things. They might travel on buses and trains independently, which is a skill that will persist for life.

Travel is our priority. It's pragmatic because it was determined that there would be no special bus to this Centre. But travel's a liberating skill. If you travel, you can get out and about, your horizons are broadened. You're not limited to a Centre, a bus, and your home. It's horrendous, how closeted mentally handicapped people can be. A spin-off from this is how closeted the public are *from* mentally handicapped people. If there were more mentally handicapped people on the buses, that would be to the greater good of all, so travel's important: it's been a great key to progress for Dee.

You asked about other priorities. When we first opened, further education was thought of as literacy and numeracy. We got pressure from parents in that respect – 'Look, so and so can't read and write. I do think it's very important. They'd get on better if they could read and write.' But for some, literacy and numeracy are peripheral: there are people in the community who hold down jobs who can't read and write at all, or very well. So now we order literacy and numeracy according to an individual student's needs. In Dee's case, we decided to push reading and writing this year.

Much more important, in terms of independence, are the kind of domestic skills we practise here. The simple meal planning and the shopping. A lot of people haven't had much experience of doing shopping and simple cooking. It's not just learning the skills, but a sense of responsibility. If things go wrong, you can't appeal to a member of staff to say, 'Why didn't you order some more soap?' Taking responsiblity is very important but that's not an easy thing to teach to young people living at home, like Dee.

Other priorities are the skills which the people develop in the group, relating with one another. It's a small group, and people have to learn how to get on, or rub along, in the same way the rest of us do. OK, you might not like someone (it's certainly not a requirement that everybody loves everybody else), but it's a requirement that people rub along together. Some mentally handicapped people are rather ego-centred, they've often been the centre of attention in the family, they haven't been out in the community very much. Dee's a good example. We do specific work in drama and movement, geared towards increasing interpersonal skills. So there's a formal approach, but a lot just happens too. In Dee's case we've concentrated on her abilities to get on with others, as you'll see from her report here.

Developing sensitivity and consideration and responsiblity to others can be fostered so that responsiblity to others develops – if it's *your* turn to cook, you must produce it. If you don't, there's a group pressure, because ten very hungry people are getting at you! Because it's a small group, a lot happens that we don't plan for – but happens because of the dynamics of that particular group. For example, you'll get a 16-year-old school-leaver behaving in a very immature fashion, and you'll hear the others saying, 'Don't do that! We're adults here, and we don't want some kid showing us up.' A lot of that just happens naturally and happily, and it relieves the staff from having to become disciplinarians.

A further priority is the way we encourage decision making. We are a self-sufficient community, we do our own shopping and cooking. There's no bulk ordering of food, so students are responsible for meal-planning, budgeting, shopping and cooking. We don't employ a gardener – and we do grow vegetables. Cleaning the Centre, domestic tasks and running the home: they need decisions about approach, timing.

Occasionally we've got to intervene – but the group does make a lot of decisions. We saw that on holiday when we were with them 24 hours a day. For example, to the extent of getting ready at 8 o'clock at night and saying: 'OK, we don't want the staff to come out with us tonight. Three of us are going into the pub, and three of us are going into this pub, and we three girls don't want to go out with the boys tonight.' To a certain extent, of course, that happens here now, but it's nice for us to see it over a 24-hour period for three weeks. And also to see that students in a foreign country (Ireland) were able to generalize what they'd learnt here (in North London).

Another priority is contact with parents. Quite often we wonder what does happen after 4 o'clock when students go home. Perhaps you've suggested that John ought to be going out in the evenings and his mum's said 'yes', but she might be very, very anxious about this and it doesn't happen. And you raise conflicts in your students – you're pushing one way and parents are pushing the other way and that's confusing. Parents must want to work with us too.

In our first year, there was an idea that you took people, put them through the course and wonderful things resulted. But nobody specified what wonderful things were going to happen, so it was quite difficult to know what one was aiming at. We're being very specific now. There was also an added problem in saying, 'All right, we'll formulate individual programmes,' but giving everybody who came a one-year fixed period here. That was a contradiction. So now we say, 'Let's look at it for three months and review it.' On occasions, people have only stayed for three months, because the referral might have been very specific. For example, 'Look, this guy is being held back, because he's not using the buses. Can you work on that?' And that's where we'll put most of our energies. More often people stay six months to two years. We develop specific programmes and report on progress under headings. Dee's Review gives an example.

Now we operate a 'roll on-roll off' system, rather than being forced to take 12 students in and get rid of 12 together. Now if we've got someone coming in who has certain behavioural problems we can begin gently, because we've got up to two years, and allow pressure to filter in – and increase when we think the person can take it. But the pressures here *are* intense. Visitors often say, 'Oh, what a cosy unit!' It is quite the reverse, really. Smallness doesn't mean cosiness. With only 12 students, everything is closely monitored, you really can't go away in a corner. But if the pressure's controlled, then it's beneficial.

### Social Development Centre
### Dee's Review

*Travel*
Dee has practised local bus routes and can try out new ones alone. She is aware of bus numbers and routes but she is not good at remembering street names. She can recognize the tube train and she knows her own station. She can use the phone and is not scared of going home at night alone.

*Sport*
She has plenty of energy, but is unfit. She has trouble balancing and has poor hand to eye co-ordination, due to a tendency to rush and panic. She should benefit from swimming: because of her individualistic nature, she is poor at team games, but is very competitive at table tennis and bowling. She is strong for her size.

*Health and Hygiene*
She is generally clean and tidy and can be fastidious. She doesn't like getting her hands dirty. Despite her obsession with germs, she has three odd habits: (1) carrying dirty tissues around; (2) wiping her nose on towels; and (3) putting sanitary towels in the wrong place.

*Clinics*

1 Dee can make her own appointment for the *dentist* but needs accompanying.

2 She has misshapen feet. She can make an appointment at the *foot clinic* and attend alone.

*Gardening*

A good worker, interested and prepared to get dirty. She can tell a diseased plant from a healthy one and understands the process of planting seeds and seeing them grow.

*Shopping*

She is efficient at self-service, but has difficulty in asking assistants for things. She can write a shopping list but rarely consults it and uses guesswork.

*Kitchen*

She has to be told to slow down and not to brandish knives! She looks dangerous, but never cuts, burns or sets herself alight – she is more of a danger to others. She is capable of common kitchen tasks and meal planning. She is conscientious about checking and testing. Her main stumbling block is timing. She cannot tell time, so has no idea of cooking times. But she can follow a simple recipe, carrying out instructions for timing by using a drawn clock face. Table laying is a problem, as there is difficulty in telling left from right.

*Clothes*

Can use launderette, but money problems are a burden. Can wash, iron, use a spin dryer and drying racks but can't sort out which clothes for which.

*House Care*

She tends to rush through a task rather than looking for results. If asked to do it again and again, she becomes efficient. She can be relied on to leave brooms, vacuum cleaners, etc., where they will be tripped over by others!!

*Social Behaviour*

She entertains at home. She is sophisticated on outings and

loves dancing. But she is hostile to and scared of men. She thinks boys are dirty and talk of sex disturbs her. She can be very flirtatious. A bit selfish regarding sharing a sweet and sharing in general.

*Discussion Group*
She would deal with criticisms of selfish attitudes by childish behaviour, or staring at the floor or walking away. Peer group pressure has little impact on her. She impresses sometimes as rather spoiled.

*Literacy*
She can read and write her name and address with no mistakes. Has childish self-image so she has developed her own book of photographs from childhood to adulthood to try to see herself in a time-sequence. She enjoyed this, worked hard at it and learned several new words as well as concepts, for example, before/after. Her speech is still monosyllabic and she gets confused by words in sentence order.

*Numeracy*
She counts up to 20 and is hazy after that. Her 1:1 correspondence is OK. She works well with small amounts of money and simple addition but she has not much idea of large amounts of money or of pricings.

12.30 Lunch

Lunch has been prepared by two of the Ashley road graduating class – beefburgers, garden peas and potatoes, followed by gooseberry fool. The alumni from Highbury Grove join in with relish and offer to help with the washing up. Dee has enjoyed her visit and the opportunity to act as tour guide. But time is passing and we hurry back to Highbury Grove to join the travel and outing group, already convened by Cathy in the library and locked in protracted negotiations about this afternoon's visit out of the Centre. The Tower of London? Camden Lock? The Horniman Museum? No. Kew Gardens. A storm is brewing – should

they go at all? These preliminary discussions and decisions
are regarded as integral to planning the outing.


2.00 Travel Group

| | |
|---|---|
| Cathy | What about you, Clive? Do you think we should go to Kew Gardens, or stay here? |
| Clive | We're going. |
| Dee | Let's go. |
| Cathy | OK, everyone wants to go, but where's Rodney? will he be outvoted when he comes, whatever he says? |
| Mike | He will, he will! |
| Cathy | Well, he's got problems. They've reorganized the 'Shop' in the afternoons and it just happens that Rod should be doing it today. OK, now *how* did we say we were going to go to Kew Gardens? |
| Dee | Train. |
| Doreen | Bus. |
| Cathy | Train or bus, so which do you think would be the quicker? |
| Dee | The train would be quicker. |
| Cathy | The train is quicker and we haven't got as much time as usual as we usually leave earlier and take our lunch. Now, if the train's the quickest and we haven't much time, what's best to go on? |
| Mike | (worried) But we haven't got no sandwiches now, have we? |
| Cathy | We don't need them today because we just had our dinner here. So if the train's the quickest and we haven't got that much time . . . |

[Rodney bursts into the room dramatically.]

| | |
|---|---|
| Rodney | I've got some very sad news for you all. |
| Cathy | Oh dear! |
| Rodney | I can't come today. |
| Mike | Oh *no*. Ohh . . . |
| Cathy | What's happening then? Are you doing the 'Shop' today? |

Rodney   Yes. [Looks sad, almost tearful.]
Cathy    Oh, we'll have to sort it out for next week, then.
         We'll talk to Sheila about it.
Rodney   [Upset] But *they* say I've got to do it next week
         and all. That I have to do it *every* Thursday. I can't
         go out with you lot, *ever*.
Cathy    Well, we'll *both* have to talk to Sheila about it
         before next week to sort it out. OK? We'll bring
         you back a postcard from Kew Gardens.
Rodney   You'll miss me!!
Cathy    We will! That's a shame but we'll sort it out by
         next week. Alright, well we'd better get coats on,
         hadn't we?

The group departed for Kew Gardens by train, mostly
coatless. The heavens opened and an August storm
descended. Eight dripping people returned at 4.00 p.m.
soaked to the skin, but happy.

## 2.30 Tea Break

An early afternoon cup of tea has been booked with Olive,
who has promised to explain the Centre's philosophy on
work. Every year some half dozen users leave Highbury
Grove Centre to move into jobs. At the same time, there is
traffic from the other direction: about six users in the Centre
have been employed temporarily in jobs outside. Jessie, an
older woman, had a cleaning job for years. The loquacious
Doreen washed dishes in a bakery. But in a recession more
users come from employment and fewer go out to jobs.

A series of work placements organized on a voluntary
basis have been arranged to give about a dozen users
selective work experience. Most of these placements are in
council-run facilities and range from a half day a week (Dee)
to two or even three days a week. (Samantha – see Friday.)

The Highbury Grove view is that fewer and fewer users
will join the paid labour force over the next twenty years. As

users will need to find opportunities to lead lives which contribute to the community, avenues outside the paid labour force need to be explored.

Certainly, mentally handicapped people say they want to work. The men usually want jobs with machines – usually cars and motor bikes – while the women express preferences for work in the caring field, usually looking after small children.

'If I left, I'd see about getting a job,' said Rodney. 'Such as, I'd love to work with the police and drive a Panda car – but I can't really drive – well, only a bumper car, that is.'

'I'd most like to work in a hospital and look after babies and children,' said Jessie.

*Olive* Well, of all the areas we've got to do something about, we have to think about a policy on work outside the Centre. We need to find more openings – volunteer or paid, even part-time. A percentage of our clients would get such satisfaction out of even half a day's work a week. They're doing something useful for other people, and they've new status. Paid work aside, the status of 'having a job' is very important – if only we could get it for them.

We need a staff member to find jobs and monitor them. We can't just sit here and say, 'Look dear, you go out there every Friday morning', and then forget it. We've got to follow up and it takes a lot of work. All kinds of problems arise. Our people are not always able to verbalize their problems; there can be misunderstandings or lack of communication for people who don't speak clearly.

The balance is not over-indulging them, but also not letting them be exploited. It's an under-developed field. At present our placements are all in council facilities: children's homes and nurseries, old people's homes. Some can't sustain stamina for more than half a day, or a day a week. But considering all the problems, outside work gives a discipline – timekeeping, appearance, hygiene. It links all the things that we do here.

## 3.00 Hostel Group

The problems of achieving the day centre *outside* the four
walls of a day centre is one difficulty. But, as we have
observed, a day centre, whether or not it has expandable
walls, only deals with its users for less than a third of the
week. Most users live with their parents, but some live in
hostels. Recently a group of hostel residents attending
Highbury Grove has been convened by Tricia, a student,
and Sheila. Their series of weekly meetings is just about to
end, but Tricia explains its origins.

*Tricia* When I first came here three months ago as a student,
the staff thought that those that lived in the hostel were very
apathetic and lethargic. One theory was that they had too
*much* social training, both at the hostel and here, and staff
wondered if they should revise their programmes. My
starting point was that I worked in a hostel elsewhere and I'd
like to exchange ideas with them about hostel life. Decision
making came up, with them feeling they were not having
much influence over what went on. If you asked them, 'Why
do you do that?' or 'Why has that happened?' or 'Why did
you choose that?' then they tended not to know. It's just the
way it was.

They complained about residents' meetings at their
hostel. Rodney said that it's alright to have these meetings
so long as something gets done after it, but they tend not to
get things done. They talked about the food, but said the
food didn't change (tinned potatoes are disgusting stuff, they
said).

So they feel that they don't have much say over their lives.
Jessie, for example, has lived in the past in her own flat. But
in the hostel her life is very confined and she gets told what's
happening and what to do. Another burning issue for them
is the question of group homes. They've been told that they
will be moved to live in these – that they'll move eventually
from a hostel to a group home. (That's part of the reason for

them being in that particular hostel, to learn how to live independently, or more independently.) But nobody seems to know what a group home is: there's a lack of understanding. No-one has showed them how it works. The descriptions they gave me varied from a cottage in the country to the staff flat at the back of the hostel! There's room for more communication between the staff of a Centre and a hostel.

## 4.00 Home

Throughout the week, it has been said repeatedly that a day centre might pose a threat to parents who wanted to view an adult mentally handicapped daughter or son as a perpetual child. In this context the staff found the views of some parents more 'retarded' than those of their children. This collision of views between staff and parents is a matter which needs more investigating: after all, as we have noted, the day centre world represents only a third of a week. What of the parents' world, the other 133 hours?

The visit to Ashley Road Centre restated the critical position of the families as an asset or an impediment to the progress of an adult mentally handicapped person. So a visit to a family seemed a good idea. As Dee's mother had agreed to meet me, Dee and I set out on the bus to the Smith family home, a grey council-owned semi-detached house quite close to the Ashley Road Development Centre.

Dee's mother had forgotten our appointment and apologized for the 'untidy' state of her immaculate house. She showed me the back garden – a riot of zinnias, carnations and dahlias. Her views were a shock. She did not want any dealing with the staff, or the Highbury Grove Centre. She did not wish to attend a parents' group. She disapproved of the way the Centre handled her daughter, to whom she referred throughout our conversation as a child.

'They don't have enough in the way of outings for the children,' she complained. But beyond this, Mrs. Smith disapproved strongly of the running of the Highbury Grove Centre. Specifically, there was no contract work for Dee, the staff had not arranged a holiday for the users, and Dee's volunteer work placement of half a day a week was not long enough. What was the point in her having more contact with the staff? – Mrs. Smith always felt uneasy at the Centre. No, she would *never* let Dee live in a hostel. What would be best for Dee would be eventually to go to live with her married sister.

In Dee's case, staff and Centre and parents and home represented two colliding worlds. For Mrs. Smith, Dee was a child who needed protection. For the Centre, Dee was an immature young woman with potential for growing up. But from the Centre's viewpoint, Mrs. Smith was either uninvolved or sabotaging of their plans. From Mrs. Smith's perspective, the staff were on the wrong track – not leaving sleeping dogs lie, trying to make silk purses out of sow's ears.

## 8.00 Parents' Meeting

That Mrs. Smith's attitude was not unique was reflected in a meeting called by the Parents' Association in the Centre that evening, where the type of programme and the values of the staff came in for both veiled and open criticism. It was clear that not all was well between the 35 hours of the week (the Centre) and the 133 hours (the home).

## 9.00 Day's End

Very few mentally handicapped people get the chance to have accelerated help such as that given by the Ashley Road Development Centre. Very few staff can achieve their own high hopes, constrained by staff shortages and ceilings in funding, as at Highbury Grove. Most centres report a gulf between the centre and parents, Dee and her mother being but one example. These issues are not minor, local problems, but a reflection of difficulties in services on a larger scale.

It is rare for centres to use their local adult education centre; a new scheme like Ashley Road Development

Centre is unique. Centres are constrained by staffing averages (the national average of staff to users of 1:9). Yet even this minimal standard is threatened by staff reductions and cutbacks. And not only Highbury Grove reports a gulf between parents and the day centre. Few centres have much contact with families, beyond the Christmas party or a summer fete.

Most day centres are confined to four walls – cut off from local world as well as from families. The most common community facilities used are the local shops and local parks. But most centres *never* use an adult education centre, only half ever use the local swimming pool or sports centre and the local library. If few mentally handicapped people get out beyond the four walls of their centre, still fewer people get in to mix with them. The centres are not the hub of community life. There is an occasional visiting member of the public, or an interested visitor or two, or maybe even a visiting social worker who comes to the Centre irregularly to discuss a case: hardly a volume of people or a type of visitor designed to make an impact on the running of a centre. So the question is: to what extent should one expect that a day centre *will* reflect the everyday world of its local community?

# Friday

## Who's Who on Friday

*Sam* is really Samantha, aged 20. She is a warm, friendly young woman with a part-time volunteer job two days a week and a range of social interests which include clothes and pop groups. She would love to be independent of her family.

*Pam* is Sam's care worker but also in charge of the Centre's outdoors activities, sports and gardening programme. She says her own experiences have made her especially aware of the need to provide channels for people's energy.

*Olive* has been introduced already as the deputy manager. She organizes the 'Weight Watch' special project, which takes place on Friday.

*Christine* manages the Highbury Grove Centre. When appointed at the age of 26, she was probably the youngest manager in the country and one of a minority of women managers. Her initial training in art was followed by the Diploma in Teaching the Mentally Handicapped. Intelligent, perceptive and committed, she is also composed, good-humoured and approachable.

*Dana* a psychologist, and *Dr. Pereira*, a psychiatrist, are visiting staff from the mental handicap hospital.

*Jim* is a breezy, self-confident salesman with enthusiasm. He is visiting the Centre to introduce a project of soft sculpture – inflatable rubber objects – as an alternative to contract work.

### 8.55 Arrival

Like half the day centres (in England and Wales at least), Highbury Grove Centre sits amidst a 'mixed' area of housing (both council and private) and light industry. Highbury is a muddle – chic Georgian houses line the park; heavy Victorian houses overhang narrow streets; small factories clutter lanes. Intractable traffic problems result from juggernauts hustling northward; an acrid smell of petrol pollution fills a clouded sky. But for all the graceless urban confusion, Highbury, like most places, offers unexpected vistas of attraction: the lightness of the Georgian houses on the park; the decorated brick in the otherwise ponderous Victorian houses, the Italian restaurant translated straight from blue Amalfi onto the Juggernaut Road.

Highbury offers a certain convenience for a day centre. Underground and overground trains, buses in profusion, parades of small shops, streets of large shops and supermarkets, fruit markets, parks, a swimming pool, libraries, churches – life itself is close at hand.

As users become less dependent on the Centre, so they become more adept at threading their way through the urban muddle outside their doorstep. Samantha is Friday's case in point. She travels alone to and from home and a voluntary work placement two days a week, attending the Centre only for three days. As she has become less dependent on the Centre, Sam's enthusiasm for attending has faded. She would dearly love to be out in the world all the time.

But first, an overview of Friday. It is the last chance to look at special projects, one old and two new. The philosophy of Highbury Grove – to be discussed later with Christine, the manager – is that innovation must be *continuous,* rather than a one-off gesture every five years. So, an 'old' project, now part of the Centre's conventional wisdom, 'Weight Watch', the Highbury Grove slimmers club, will be visited. Mid-morning will be spent with the gardeners, a project established about six months ago to take care of the outside of the Centre. And this afternoon, the newest project of all, the soft sculpture rubber 'inflatables', promoted by Jim.

Today is the opportunity to uncover the philosophy and to integrate the threads. Meeting Christine, we will discuss the

Centre's aims, methods of achieving its timetable, its philosophy on appointing staff, the way it sets about assessments and its managerial structure. This implies that 'it' (the Centre) has a life of its own. But 'it' is not the sum total of staff. More likely, it is the alchemy of all the members, staff and users, of the Centre. It is 'they' who breathe life into and infuse 'it', rather than 'it' directing them.

## 9.00 Care Group

Exactly 9.00 a.m., Samantha (known as Sam) introduces herself with charm. Born with Down's syndrome, she is now a bubbly 20-year-old who lives with her parents, three brothers and sisters. Last year, she spent six months at 'Ashley Road' and she now (amongst other things) can count to a hundred, write simple short stories, read packet labels and cook a simple meal. I have been told that Sam is normally bright, cheerful and sociable, but this morning, she takes some coaxing to believe that she has anything to offer our discussion. However, once the tape-recorder starts, she confides as follows:

*Sam* I'm very independent now. I'd like to get a full-time job. I'd like to live in a flat. I can travel alone, I go to work by myself three days a week on the 37 bus. I can get myself a meal and do my room. I like my job at the nursery. I play with the babies and change their nappies and help out. I enjoy child care. I'd like to get married, but I don't think I'd want to have a child. Yes, I might change my mind, but I don't think so.

I think I should leave the Centre now, I'm so independent. My mum and dad are going to move out of London when my dad retires. I'd like to move into a flat with other girls, I don't want to go with my parents.

I like music. I go to a folk club in Birmingham once a month. I do sing a lot – there's five other girls in our group –

the Black Diamonds. And there's three lads. So that's five, six, seven, eight, nine. Nine in the group. I love it.

Sam goes to rejoin the care group meeting, which takes place in a Social Education room with Pam as her care worker. Because Sam is so 'advanced' she spends a relatively long period of time at each activity: long periods at one activity to develop concentration is the key to understanding her programme format. Today, she will spend most of the day working on the horticulture project with Pam, who is also her care worker. Sam produces her timetable and explains it herself.

| | Today is *Friday* | *Monday* | *Tuesday* | *Wednesday* | *Thursday* |
|---|---|---|---|---|---|
| **Sam's Programme** | | | | | |
| AM | Gardening | Social education (literacy/ numeracy) | Work project (nursery) | Sports Centre and independent travel | Work project (nursery) |
| PM | Free choice (gardening) | Social education (literacy/ numeracy) | Work project (nursery) | Free time | Work project (nursery) |

But before Sam goes to garden she dashes off to the 'weigh in' with the 'Weight Watch' group. After she disappears, Pam discusses whether Sam had improved in her time at the Centre.

*Pam* Oh yes, Sam has come on ever so well. Two years ago, her mother wouldn't let her travel outside the home alone and she certainly wouldn't let her cook. In fact, she even used to bathe Sam and she was quite unhappy about her having sex instruction at the Centre. Now she travels alone, cooks for herself and bathes herself and washes clothes. Sex instruction is still a problem. But as a result of her acceleration at Ashley Road, Sam feels quite frustrated with life at this Centre. She does not find being here as satisfying as being at her work placement. Sam would like to leave altogether, although at present her parents wouldn't approve.

We sorted out some new priorities for Sam when we held the annual review last year. Handling money was a problem for her, so was taking responsibility for her own hygiene. She was ready to develop more complex domestic skills beyond tea-making and can-opening. To help implement these things we suggested the following targets for the next six months: targets which were agreed to by Sam's parents.

### Targets for Sam

First, Sam is to make tea on Sunday for the whole family.

Second, Sam should wash her own pants and tights out each night.

Third, Sam is to practise her own hairwashing at the Centre (she has trouble washing the back of her head).

Fourth, Sam is to increase her number of hours at volunteer work, since this is what she most enjoys – and she has been a success.

Sam's become more practical and down to earth in the last year. Before that she was frequently in a dream world, a fantasy world, really believing that she was a pop star, for instance, and being very moody, sullen and difficult. She seems to have got some help from the discussions in the Wednesday group, the video group that became a talking group. Once or twice she'd go off into her fantasies, but very rarely. She almost grew to be the person she was in the group, rather than the moody person she was around the place. Or maybe it's just that she's grown up suddenly.

## 9.30 *'Weight Watch'*

This group of about 20 voluntary members meets on Friday with Olive. Those with other engagements (such as Sam), who need to get to the garden, get priority on the scales.

*Olive*   It's a question of people being aware of their shape, their posture and how they look. We try to give an idea that they can look other than a great lump. It has changed people drastically – their motivation and their awareness and how they can cope with life. Most do well: only a few have hardly any response at all. It's based on an awareness of foods that are healthy. Certainly not being rigid about diet – no counting calories, or anything like that – it's awareness of what is healthy. That you *can* live without cakes and biscuits and chips and fatty things. Well, how have you found it, Sam? What kind of foods have you found that you do best on?

Sam       Salads, eggs, greens, meat and gravy.
Olive     And what sort of things do you try not to eat?
Sam       I try not to eat potatoes, or cake, or biscuits or chips.

Life at the Centre used to be handing around the sweeties. You came in with something in your pocket and all day you were handing around, or having a sweet in between. 'Weight Watch' is voluntary but it's become a status symbol to belong. They are their own policemen; they keep an eye on each other! Sweets, cakes and doughnuts brought in to go with their tea just disappeared altogether. A way of life changed. People were more comfortable and looked better. They felt more able to go out and about. Their clothes looked more beautiful. they could go into a shop and look at things and see how they would fit.

Originally I employed all kinds of methods to encourage it – first, weekly rewards of fruit drinks and fruit jellies from gelatine. Then I wound that down so that we had rewards only at the end of term, or for a great event, for somebody doing tremendously well – reaching the two or three stone they've lost. Second, we had charts and photographs to take home. They would be pictured on the rowing machine, or the bicycle, or skipping. Third, we used to have scrapbooks – and paste things, pictures of food that were healthy and unhealthy, things that you mustn't eat, or only eat occasionally. We've gone through the gamut, over the years, of all kinds of ideas. But the result is that, when you come into the Centre now, you don't see fat people. Only fat newcomers: we've got about two really difficult cases. The whole reward system has become unnecessary – they get their reward when they look into this full-length mirror.

It is a three-way thing, the person themselves, first; the back-up of the family, second; and the back-up here, third. They are all important but the family is crucial. When the family's not concerned, or where they think it's natural that their daughter be thirteen stone, there's no response.

A record book, entered every week, they take home and proudly show, or otherwise. Also 'Weight Watch' is regular, it must be every week at the same time, and every week without fail. As you see, they don't have to be encouraged to come – they are all here, waiting. But it has to be self-motivated. Doreen says that it doesn't matter that she is thirteen stone. Yet she must feel the odd one out because she is enormous. She's new, she works in a bakery in the evenings, has chips every day. I said, 'Of course, it's up to you to decide. What you want to look like is up to you. But if you want to look like so and so, then you've got to, for a while, cut out the things which are fattening.' So it has to always be self-motivated.

We also have 'wasters' who need to put their weight up. Well, take Timothy, who never remembers what day it is. Yet he was down here earlier and weighed in first. He's a very damaged soul, but he is keen to put his weight up. Some haven't got much appetite, but once they realize that they are at risk if they are so thin, they tend to be more

willing to try things and try and eat a little bit more and eat
things that are a little more fattening like ice-creams.

Sam   Well, I *never* eat ice-creams. I have apples, oranges,
      pears, grapes. Only fruit!
J.C.  Only fruit! You sound as if you eat very sensibly. Do
      you like coming to Weight Watch yourself?
Sam   Yes, I do! I like keeping my weight down and getting
      weighed every Friday. So that I don't put on. I feel
      better. [Sam, formerly overweight, now merely
      solid, disappears.]

*Olive*  Our biggest success was fifteen stone eight and was
four foot nine. Barbara is now nine stone six. So she's lost
six stone over four years. Her mother said, 'Oh she'll never
lose weight.' We were worried about her as we'd lost two
girls who died through heart attacks in that very unusual
summer heat. A doctor prescribed some tablets and then
Barbara began to lose weight. At this stage we asked
mothers of the very difficult ones if they'd like to join in.
She's changed her way of life. Before, mother said 'Oh,
she's got to have her little Mars Bar, she can't be without
anything' implying that the Mars Bars were the be-all and
end-all of the girl's pleasure! We explained that she'd have
no pleasure at all in life – in fact she was 'at risk' in life itself
– if she didn't change.

  Posture is very important – we don't do enough. One or
two, especially those who have lost weight and are thin, are
very round-shouldered. They do posture in the movement
classes, but it's also something to highlight and tie up at
'Weight Watch'. 'Weight Watch' also relates to exercise and
sports. Discussing with every person what they're going to
eat on the weekend. Some sit all weekend, behind their
curtains, with their taperecorder, or their records, from
Friday to Monday morning. Now with constant discussion
you *can* suggest they ask to go out, to walk to places, to go to
the park, if you've an animal or dog, to take it out for a
walk. Individual discussion is crucial.

See that chart from the Health Education Council? Individuals choose an exercise they like best, put that chart up in their bedroom and they can follow the diagrams. 'Which one do you like best?' 'Let's see how you do it?' 'Would you like to copy such and such?' It's all very simple – there's nothing complicated or clever about how to encourage that. It's the whole thought process which is so stimulating.

Now let's weigh people. Barbara, you're first. Now, Barbara is going on holiday soon and she's dieting on cottage cheese and salad, with melons and grapefruit. [Weighs in Barbara.]

That's fantastic, nine stone four! Fifteen and a half stone down to nine stone four. The thing is now, whenever Barbara wants to go on a binge, or goes up to her sister's place and has a big meal, that's OK, because she knows now how to lose it again. It's in her pattern of life – to eat less, and she knows what to eat. She knows what kinds of foods are fattening.

Now she can walk up steps without getting breathless and she's gone down two sizes in trousers! It was mainly a matter of stopping her eating biscuits non-stop. I said to her mother, 'Why do you buy them? If she can't resist them, don't have them in the house. Give her other things that she likes – don't have biscuits.' She lost two stone right away, just by giving up biscuits! She was a fiendish biscuit eater! Now she has one biscuit now and again as a treat.

## 10.30 Coffee Talk

Whilst Olive starts weighing in Linda (down six stone and now a runner and a cycler) Christine nods her head around the door. Seizing the opportunity of an uninterrupted ten-minutes talk, we take coffee to her office. Today, Christine looks almost Pre-Raphaelite, a figure in a Burne-Jones painting. She wears a long skirt and a flowing white blouse; blonde hair falls down her back. One would be unwise to take this romantic appearance at face value; her manner is businesslike and her mind disciplined and tough.

*Christine* On paper, we've got individual programmes but we haven't achieved it in practice. Everybody's week has been individually planned. But the significance of what they achieve in each session isn't yet individual enough for it to be always beneficial. The problem with a given staff ratio is how you work out what *activities* you should be doing that link directly to the *needs* of the person, without going to the file every day to look up the needs in detail. So every staff member has to hold in his or her head an awful lot of information about each user. Just imagine, in one session, you've got seven other people, all with different needs, then in the next session, you'll have another seven!

How do you move your knowledge of that *need* around the Centre? How do you move around different activities and therefore staff? For example, if your aim is to teach what we call positional values ('on', 'up' or 'under') – it is very boring to be repetitive and to keep doing that in a classroom. Our aim is to teach in a number of different situations. So Leanne would be asked in the craft room to put paint *on* the paper; back in the Special Needs room to put the cup *under* the sink.

How do we move that area for Leanne and others around the Centre, between all the different staff, without having massive discussions, daily, on seventy people? How do you get all the staff to know what every single person *needs* as relates to their own areas of *skill*? Once we achieve *that*, then we have individual programmes!

Then, how do we get on with the task in hand within our present staff ratio? We could set loads more objectives for different individuals, but there are only so many staff. It's frustrating to watch jobs just go by the board because you're dashing around after too many people. So at times it's disorganized. It would be nice to pick up what others are thinking by thought transference! It's good though to have other members of staff working with one person. It must be awful, working with the same person for the whole week. Other people pick up things you're not picking up, or perhaps someone else will find a better way of getting something over.

Then, of course, not all staff are equally skilled in all areas, so you can't expect them to achieve equally with the same person.

It's difficult to describe the aims of the Centre without coming out with pat statments to do with 'developing the individual's potential' and that sort of thing (which has nothing to do with the individual!). We're here to offer something to people who are so varied, so complex, that we need to look at the Centre as a place that offers a *varying* service – of different types, of different natures – to quite different people. So I see this Centre as a service, which offers something to individuals which is neither restrictive, nor containing, but developing and expressive. It varies between maximum care and maximum support (as in Special Needs) to minimum care, but maximum support for people about to leave us (like Sam).

This means that as a Centre we have to change, according to who we have at a particular time. And we're also part of a much bigger whole; we're not isolated; we use other services – the social services department as a whole, further education, the health service, social security, careers officers, employment officers, schools, residential care workers, group homes, sports centres, parents, and what have you.

To sum up, our aim is *individual* service to people, a service that isn't restrictive or containing, a service that practises allowing a person to express and to develop himself or herself. The traditional work ethic for mentally handicapped people is restrictive, because it's not taking into account what a person needs to develop. The work ethic can be very effective if somebody *needs* training *in that area*, but usually it is just a routine which has lost its value.

## 11.00 Gardening

Sam and Pam make their way to the spare and unyielding-looking space outside the Centre at the back. There is a greenhouse, but there is a big job of development to be done. To use this barren plot, Pam aims to invite people to take responsibility for helping to maintain the garden as part of the Centre. Inside, Council cleaners do toilets and classrooms; kitchen staff prepare meals. The garden is one area where members of the Centre are completely responsible for planning and maintenance.

*Pam* Yes, the garden has got to be maintained; if you develop one part and totally neglect the rest, it's overrun before you can turn around. But we want to get people into the seasonal rhythm of gardening. We propagate in winter, cultivate and then move seedlings off to the greenhouse and put them in frames until they're big enough for people to see that they're cauliflowers or lettuces. Then we plant out.

But going back to the maintenance work, we've drawn up a huge wall chart, using photographs. The gardeners can go back to the chart, the photographs are all laid out. For instance, in mowing grass, we look at the chart. This says the first job is to pick up stones off the grass; second, put them in a bucket; third, empty the bucket; fourth, wash out the bucket; fifth, you get out the actual lawnmower. 'Please mow the grass' – that's your job. But there are an awful lot of steps to doing what seems a simple job.

The hardest job is weeding. I have problems explaining weeding; you can't say, 'Well, this is a weed and this is a plant.' When you ask what gardening's all about, ninety per cent say 'digging'. Digging a hole, not quite knowing why, is what they relate to gardening.

When I first started, a group of people wanted to do gardening. They seem to feel close to the earth. It's good for them, if that's how they relate to their time here. They're very enthusiastic. They get an awful lot of enjoyment, that's how you notice it. They're keen and ready to go. It's very practical; you can actually cut out talking and show them what to do. Some of these people, they're London-born and bred the same as me and perhaps never have had a garden.

The ones that don't want to do it show up quite clearly. You have to persuade them that it's a nice thing to do. This year, the soil was pretty rough, as you can see. So we planted a variety of things, to see what was going to take. We've been lucky. I don't think it's a marvellous crop but at least they can pick a strawberry this summer – although some say they're grapes.

[Pam moves back to the gardeners, who say they need a drink; the sun is hot. After lemonade all round, the dirty horticulturalists get back to watering, weeding and a spot of digging. I have asked Pam if we can discuss how she came to work at the Centre. Pam was built to be a sports person – tall and broad-shouldered. Yet she is softly spoken, very gentle and empathic.]

I was given a chance to work here, two and a half years ago. I started off working in the kitchen, but as soon as I'd finished my work I'd be outside playing games and talking to people. I became a care assistant, then progressed to a care officer.

But it's been a struggle. I came to Highbury Grove to prove myself. I wanted to use my talents on sports and games to relate to people who are underprivileged and don't fit in – oddballs. They need to be treated like growing plants; not like shit. I have a special feeling for the people here, as I was brought up in care, in a kid's home, from about six weeks to eight years old, and that affected my life. I went through the courts, mental institutions. When I was about fourteen, building up, I was expelled from school. I had a huge chip on my shoulder that it was everybody else – it was society in general, it wasn't me.

I went through a psychiatric hospital for two years, and a day centre [for the mentally ill]. I had quite a lot of dealings with the local social services department; I demanded an awful lot of them. I was using the day centre as a prop – if I didn't get it I'd smash the place up. Then I spent ten months in Henderson Hospital, quite an ordeal. You had to be quite tough to go through with everything. It became clearer, the way my family were setting me up as the scapegoat and the whole cycle of what was happening. Yes? In a way – I was carrying out a role for society too. It's really weird, but even at school, they *needed* somebody like *me* to act out. It became very clear. I'd become the individual that they'd created, yes?

Then I worked in a youth club, part time. I really enjoyed the work and found that I could relate to young people. That's why I came to work here at Highbury Grove. I had to prove myself and I was given a chance. Christine knew my background and she was the only person prepared to give me this chance. It's been a struggle.

I no longer feel resentful about my past, because it's why I am what I am now. I'm happy being me – not split up into little pieces – I feel quite whole. All my experiences are valuable, if I can use them. I have to be careful not to over-identify with people here because that's not doing them any favours. Empathy yes, that's important and valuable. Not many people actually know how it feels to be an outsider. As I said, I'm very sensitive when we go swimming, and they're slow and you hear the lady behind the counter say 'Oh God. Just as well we haven't got a queue.' It makes me feel angry, I can imagine what it does to them, when you hear such snide remarks. They are rejected, there's no two ways about it.

This work is rewarding, it makes you feel that you've achieved something, so that means they give you something nice back. I don't know how to put this as I'm not too clear about it myself; I get, not so much a sense of importance, but a sense that I feel worthwhile. I've felt totally worthless, and good for nothing apart from scrubbing floors. I have actually got a brain but I had to convince myself, and that's what gave me the energy to go on. And again, you see, what's why I get the idea of channelling people's *energy* here into games and gardens! I don't go and pester social services now and I don't smash places up. Because I've got something I enjoy doing and hopefully I've got something to give.

12.00 Christine's Office – Staff

I am here to ask Christine to discuss the Centre's policy on the recruitment of staff and how the staff group, as a team, work together.

*Christine*   Over the past five years the original staff, except one, have left. It's been gradual. But now ( and looking at how one changes a Centre) every member of staff has been selected by me. Now we all work pretty much in tune, towards similar things.

But a lot don't know what it's like to work in work centres or other day centres, therefore they don't know that there's a battle! The danger is that development could stop. It's odd to have worked through a fight and come to the place where it could stop, because people don't see how *crucial* it is to keep moving. As long as staff are not *quite* satisfied (providing they're happy, but not satisfied), we can still move in a positive way. (Dissatisfied in that they can't do everything they want to do. And that they don't always see the value in their work.)

In recruiting staff, I think about what the Unit needs. First, I look for skills. For our last appointment, we needed somebody who knew more about educational development that anybody else. Next, I expect people to be hardworking, in a physical sense. I don't want people who are just thinkers, they need to be doers as well – that's very important. And third, people need to be committed and enthusiastic. So, they need to have some skills, to be hardworking, and to be committed to their job. Even if the commitment's only going to be for a limited time, for three or six months, I need to depend on them for that period. I guess those three qualities are difficult to find in interviews, quite honestly! Recruiting staff is frightening. It's very difficult to get rid of them, if they're not very good.

It's very difficult to find people who can actually do the job well, and be innovative too, not static. It's particularly difficult to recruit from mental handicap itself, from people who have the specified training. Staff from other day units for the mentally handicapped want to pull us back all the time.

It's important to have an age range for staff, just as we do for clients. I tried recently to recruit an older member of staff, male and middle-aged. I couldn't find anybody, presumably because of the poor pay. It is easier to recruit people who are a bit younger, because of the pay. People who change jobs and want to move in different directions. Generally that seems to happen a lot in the late twenties – those who have developed some sort of conscience. That is another difficulty, you have to sift out those who've developed a social conscience that's only going to last a couple of weeks! And then there's another group to beware, those who are looking for an easy life!

Young staff need support. As manager, I need support too. I begin to fear that I might become the static manager! Twenty odd years ago, innovators became static, because they didn't move on with the times. Every time I say in a staff meeting, 'No I'm not going to have that', I think, 'Is that a good idea I just threw out?' But the attitude matters more than age. I think about what people have to offer, if they can do the job that's there, if they are willing to look at their own restrictions and limitations and to perhaps work on those. Or to admit them and say, 'no, I can't do that, could somebody else?'

Not everybody has to be open all the time. I'm not, and I don't expect anybody else to be. For example, I don't accept people having had a bad night before and taking this out on the clients next morning – that's not openness, that's self-indulgence. I think you should put on a good face while you're at work. That contradicts in many ways lots of my other views but equally I don't mind that contradiction, because we do get paid to do a job of work.

You can go to centres where they are so open as to be destructive – staff end up looking at themselves so much that they're forgetting about the job they have been paid to do. It's good to look at yourself, but if you really need to do it desperately, in a great deal of depth, go somewhere else and do it in you own time!

You must have a pride in yourself if you're going to take on a job in this field. You must give as much as you expect to take. Staff can give a lot and can take back absolutely nothing. A manager has to put an awful lot of support in to prevent that. It's absolutely exhausing for somebody to work with someone eight hours a day for a year, just to have them say, 'fuck off', as they're walking out of the door. On the other hand, if you work with somebody for a year, and they blossom to do some little thing, you need to have the eyes to see that as a beautiful and rewarding thing for the whole year. I think that's another part of my job, to make sure that people do see those things and do get as much joy out of them as they possibly can. Because otherwise the job can be really, to be honest, a bit – ugh!

I see my job as a facilitator, Someone who is supportive of staff who are having to undergo quite drastic changes all the time. And perhaps, as an innovator. But my concern is to be supportive to the staff, and assist them to work through their day-to-day existence with their groups, where they're taking them and what they want to do. I was going to say instigating change and making new directions, but this has changed. Staff are now so innovative, moving themselves very rapidly and readily and the direction they're moving in is so very good, that I no longer have a fight to fight!

I did have a battle at the beginning. It's easier in many ways with something to fight for! Now, sometimes I end up thinking, 'Oh God, I should be thinking of something really new!!' Yet, for the time being, my main job can only be supportive. I can only inject ideas here, there and everywhere. If people are working with particular groups of clients all the time, they lack an overview and so I can inject ideas in that way. That allows me to still hang onto the job of being innovative, to a certain extent!

## 12.30 Lunch

At lunch, we are joined by three visiting members of staff; a psychologist, a psychiatrist, and a community nurse. Early this afternoon there is to be an assessment clinic and for these occasions the staff of the Centre are joined by an outside team from the mental handicap hospital of the local health authority. This hospital, Harperbury, is actually outside London, in Hertfordshire. But despite the exigencies of distance the recent collaboration between hospital and day centre has been very fruitful. For Dana, the psychologist working in the hospital, the day centre has opened up the community dimension of her work. She is encouraged to try programmes which would not be accepted by the more conservatively-minded hospital staff. She is able to bring to the Centre a detailed appreciation of the way to calculate the limits imposed by handicaps and the range of movement that might be expected of a user in a given time. For Dr Pereira, the day centre is an appropriate London base to follow up his outpatients. By seeing his patients at the day centre rather than the hospital, he can sometimes, he says, prevent lengthy admissions to hospitals by judicious offering of occasional and respite care, and his information about patients is greatly enhanced by being able to meet day centre staff.

This leads into the topic of how Highbury Grove goes about assessing its users. Christine reminds us that when she became manager, five years ago, there were no records about clients and no reviews. To get a system going required thought.

*Christine* Conventional textbook assessments were too restrictive. It said where somebody had got up to and gave you a baseline. But none of us could get the next stage together at all! It was far too generalized and it didn't aid in developing programmes. As of five years ago, the staff were untrained: they'd all worked supervising contract work. It was all very well for me to say, 'OK, you're all going to embark on Social Education programmes.' But without being in the groups all the time, working with them, showing them what it meant and where it was supposed to be going, it was impractical.

We had to develop an assessment which would do more than assess the client needs and give baselines. It needed to be more positive. It didn't need to say, 'This person is functioning at this level', but instead, 'This is where this person could be going' and 'This is how you get there.' So it was important for staff as well as client development. We spent time working on that: it brought staff together. We had a week's workshop to develop our own assessment and how we'd see it (see Appendix II).

At the same time, I introduced outside staff like psychologists and psychiatrists into the Centre as supportive to the staff and to help us with the assessments. Also to aid work with clients and how you programmed them. So, the whole change was coming at the same time. The gears were going at different speeds, some were very slow, some faster.

At present, we've had to put annual assessments back into slow gear. They're essential but time-consuming to prepare. Until we get more staff there's no point in defining new needs in the clients. We devote a half day to each client, invite parents to come in and have our psychologist and psychiatrist here. As you have already seen, a great deal of our work flows from the annual assessment; it's vital we keep up to date.

## 2.00 Inflatables

Whilst I am reflecting that this is a Centre where staff, as well as users, are encouraged to develop their abilities, I am reminded that it's time to join the project known as 'inflatables'. Jim runs a project sponsored by the Mental Health Foundation and his mission is to take his enthusiasm and his rubbery objects to day centres. He is working at Highbury Grove Centre with six selected users (Rodney and Clive are two of the six) for a fortnight.

It is hard to describe Jim's inflatables in words: they are to be felt rather than described. They are large movable pieces of soft sculpture – huge balloons or sausages or kite shapes which are made of tough, red, yellow or blue rubber. They are measured out, shaped, glued and inflated. And then? Jim explains for himself.

*Jim* First, what I try to achieve is something for the mentally handicapped individuals to do. Their confidence is built up so they can tackle larger things saying, 'Oh, I'll have a think about that', rather than, 'No I'm not capable.' A lot of this group lack confidence. We haven't reached their ability limit. Second, we are giving something to society, something wanted. We take the 'inflatables' out of the Centre, say to a playground, or a children's home, or an Event. In those circumstances, we are the best adverts for the mentally handicapped. People say, 'Oh, I like that.' 'That pleases me.' 'I want more of that.' So the peculiarity is that some 'normal' people in our society say they want to see more of the mentally handicapped because when they are out demonstrating inflatables they are the people that are returning energy into the community and improving the vitality of life, if you like. You've made a profit, but not a monetary profit, an energy profit.

At an Event, we'll deal with a crowd of twenty thousand or a group of five. When you first take out a group, you protect it. That is, you start in your own centre, then you might go out to a school. (Maybe the school they came from, which is quite nice for them. 'Hello teacher, look what I'm doing now,' and all that.) Then you just keep building up confidence from easy jobs to hard jobs. You *could* just sit there and pick your nose all day long, or you could treat it as a cottage industry, gradually become the managing director, taking decisions like, 'Do we want to go to Fred Nerk's school on a Saturday? How do we get there? How much does it cost? Insurance?' You can, if you've got the ability, get up to be managing director, but you can fit in the industry anywhere you like – as stock controller, maintenance person, anything.

Centres have to get away from the idea of making money in contract work and look to projects which can put these people back into society. The idea of getting mentally handicapped people out into factories is Victorian. There are three million people out there who don't have any work already, because their factory has shut down.

I'm opposed to contract work. You've seen it! I was at a Centre the other day and they're making nine million bottle

tops. Even *I* couldn't make money out of it, the small rates
they're being paid – even if I worked flat out, *I* couldn't
make money. Contract work is outdated: it started abut 100
years ago with the idea that the mentally handicapped, or
loonies, or whatever – could do something – and it's grown
up in the years to contract work. Meanwhile outside
everyone's becoming unemployed. There's no work about,
there's a new technology. But in some centres they've just
now got up to the concept of contract work!

So what we in centres have got to do is take a couple of
jumps in front of everyone else. While the main society
sorts out unemployment, we can jump in front. That is,
we're working to give people satisfaction with their leisure
time. It's working leisure, people in the future will be paid
for leisure. So I want to be a pioneer – to put the mentally
handicapped in front of the 'normal'.

My problem is that I could go in to a centre and give
them the whole earful, but then the department of social
services turns around and might say 'Well, look, if you
were to make some money for us, we'd let you do it.' But
they could not make inflatables at monetary profits. I know
one centre up in the north that takes real pride in that it
makes more money than another unit. So they didn't like
me, because my project wasn't going to make them much
money. But then they realized that the things I was making
were very popular – so their unit was going to make money
after all. And I would say, 'That's not the point.' If I want
to make inflatables profitably, then I'd employ 'normal
people', or so-called normal people – more able people
than this group here, for instance. Then I would sit there,
five days a week, working myself to death, but making a
load of money. A funny thing is that centres still do think
that way. They say, 'Money – oh!' And when I say, 'Well,
why don't you just *do* it?' they say, 'We've got to make
money.'

Work in centres shouldn't be devised just to keep people
occupied! Alright, if it was in normal industry it wouldn't
be to keep them occupied, it would be for them to make

money. At the end of the week, the workers would go down to the pub and get their brain back again.

If you've ever worked at something that makes people happy yourself, you know how you get an enormous buzz out of that. So when this group finishes its first inflatable, you come and see their faces then! they'll all be saying, 'Oh, I made that', 'We all want that.' There's nothing abnormal about that, we all need to be wanted, and the rest of it. So contract work, all it does is keep down riots or whatever! But this isn't a zoo, it's a day centre!

I do think some centres are changing. This one is a good example. It was a contract-work centre five years ago. There's a need for creators of ideas; but you also need the sellers of ideas like me, to spread them through the countryside.

## 3.00 On Social Change

With issues of social change in mind, I return to Christine's office to ask her how the change from the contract-work centre of the past to the Highbury Grove of today was achieved.

*Christine* When I took this job five years ago, I was in a hostel. Day centres were locked places down the road. Nobody visited; residents used to come home and complain. I never actually saw a day centre because we weren't allowed in! So when I went to the day centre (which wasn't in this particular building), the first thing that struck me was how repressed and quiet the people were and how dark and dismal the place was.

My first concern was just to open it up. Like opening doors and having the place painted. Like livening things up a bit, and saying, 'You don't have to feel hemmed in here.' It was so dark and dull and dismal, I felt bad about that. How could somebody go to a place like that, all the time?

The clients were quiet and repressed and just *sitting*, doing really boring things. It wasn't only that, but they were being totally exploited. That offended me. They were packing ring-boxes. I can't remember the exact cost but I think they were paid something like ten pence a gross. And these boxes were stacked to the ceiling in the limited space! We should have been charging the businessman miles, miles more than what he was paying us for packing them, even just in storage. He was using us as a free storage bay – and that incensed me. Apart from being a ratepayer, I felt that handicapped people were being exploited, and here I was, sitting back and watching it. So exploitation was one of the first things to get rid of.

That was an internal battle for me. I couldn't say we'd get rid of the contract work overnight, because our old building was so limited in space that you couldn't offer new activities to people. And I didn't want people sitting around doing nothing all day. (It is better to do repetitive work, perhaps, than to do absolutely nothing.) So I couldn't just throw it out. We had to gradually introduce different activities, to build up on what we could reasonably do, given the building and facilities. Which meant moving people out of the Centre too.

We moved people out into different services, into Colleges of Further Education, into Adult Education. People started to move through the four walls. The battle was taking on the status quo, the staff attitudes, the building. The problem was how you fitted all those elements together and produced something better. Sometimes, if you do have a bad lot, it is quite useful because you've got something to fight against. So it's often easier to be clearer about where you're going, when you've got a battle. When you haven't, the issues can become blurred.

The other thing was an assumption of 'them and us'. When I first came I used to assume that I would run the place without taking into account what mentally handicapped people feel they need. But if the clients weren't here, we wouldn't have a job anyway, so in fact they call the shots. The people who attend here *are* people, just as much as we are. OK, they have some different needs (I'm not so sure they are all that different, anyway) – but nevertheless they *are* people and I've got no right to say that I can contain and restrict one of them, any more than they've got that right over me! I have a responsibility to ensure that they're as *safe* as possible and as *happy* as possible. But they have that responsibility towards me as well.

The reality outside the Centre is that there is a sort of 'them and us' thing. There *is* class structure; it would be rather nice if there wasn't. But why should I set up a mini-version of that in the Centre when I've got the possibility of not doing it?

When I took the job half the staff wanted to change, but half didn't. My problem was how to make the changes, taking into account that some people needed direction and some felt they didn't. The staff had been directed for many years, as well as the clients. I couldn't get any consensus on where to move. So I ended up having to tell people to change and then working through it afterwards. It wasn't the least bit democratic at the time. You couldn't expect people who had taken orders for ten years just to change overnight.

On paper, we *do* have a hierarchy here. I am responsible *to* somebody in the headquarters of the social services department and the staff are responsible to me, so we do have quite a rigid structure. But it's how we present that structure and how we blur the edges! How we interpret the system, to prevent it being restrictive. Yes, there is a hierarchy but it's how you operate it that counts. You can't make totally free decisions, mainly because you can't come on and say that you want people to be happy and learn things and then put them at risk. *That* would be restrictive.

Sometimes it has been levelled at me that I am too hierarchical and dogmatic! But we discuss how viable it is to maintain a hierarchy. Whilst I feel some safety in being officer in charge, the staff do as well, because they can always use that if something is going quite wrong. If it's used too often of course it won't work.

This place is very highly structured; not to maintain a hierarchy, but to ask for detailed participation. The skill I most need from the staff is maintaining that high degree of participation in the structure without making it restrictive. A lot of centres have the hierarchy, and operate a system where the manager is in charge and staff have very little say. Yet they don't have any structure at all for the clients! So they have a layer of a hierarchy on top, as a veneer, but they forget completely about everybody else.

I found that the clients had set up a structure for themselves. They had 'lower-grade' people whom they didn't talk to and 'higher-grade' people whom they aspired to be. Now, all the clients are highly timetabled and structured, so they know exactly what they're doing (or should do), where they're going. But within each bit of the structure it allows some self-expression and they have some choice within that programme.

We want to make everyone feel good about what they're doing and everyone makes efforts to make it appear that the structure itself is willing to change. When you develop that situation, people aren't static. So you don't say, 'Sam goes to social training every Monday to learn such and such a skill for the next two months.' Obviously one doesn't put a time restriction on it, she has to go into that area to learn something for a period of time. but once she's learned that, then you've got to change that particular bit of structure. So you've got to be constantly moving.

## 3.30 Party Afternoon

On Friday everyone has a free choice. As a user you can choose to join Cathy at embroidery, John at printing, or Sheila at drama. Occasionally a care group has a special get-together in the late afternoon. Sam has a birthday tomorrow, so her care group are having a do; someone has organized a birthday cake and brought in some records. Christine and I decide to gatecrash – with reinforcements of orange juice. Over the strains of Abba, I shout at Sam:

J.C.   Happy birthday, Sam. Are you singing with your group this weekend?

Sam   Yes! This club we go to, in Birmingham, I go there once a month.

J.C.   To Birmingham? All that way? Who do you go with?

Sam   A person who used to be leader of our club is in a record company. I do sing a lot.

J.C.   Do you really? Do you enjoy that?

Sam   I do. But I shall *shake* an awful lot. I really *shake*. You should come to see me on stage. It really pulls me about!

We attack the birthday cake and pull that about. Good luck to Sam and her group; her wish to live in a flat; her efforts towards more efficient hairwashing and delicious Sunday teas!


## 4.00 Afterword

This account of everyday life at Highbury Grove is of course selective. We have not had time to go on an outing, to visit the Sports Centre, to go to the theatre, to spend time in a kitchen craft or cooking class, to spend a morning at a job placement, to visit the physiotherapy or movement session, or to sit in the needlework group. We have not met all the staff and we have only got to know five of the seventy users well.

Highbury Grove Centre, it has been made clear, is far from being a typical day centre. It has been chosen as the subject of this book precisely because it is not typical. But neither is it so atypical as to have nothing to say to other settings which care for mentally handicapped people. The staff at Highbury Grove work with less than favourable staff ratios; with extremely difficult clients and sometimes disapproving parents, with the odd staff member who considers the whole enterprise to be misguided. But despite all, Highbury Grove has managed to change itself – its changes have not been imposed by higher authorities from outside the Centre.

To put it in social science language, this has been a case study documenting the changes in one organization through the eyes of the members of the organization itself. It has been about changing a hierarchical, non-participative management structure into a more collective, participative form; about changing a programme where clients fitted into the routine of the organization to a programme where the routine is secondary to meeting the individually defined needs and rights of each client. But above all, this study has been about the use of time; time as the servant and the tool rather than as master and tyrant.

# End

The previous chapters have described good times and bad times for Leanne, Clive, Paul, Dee and Sam. Whether they were up against time, with enough time, or even when there was time to spare, time was an asset as well as a liability. The timetable was a constructive tool; time-honoured ways of doing things were altered and the slow-motion world of these mentally handicapped people was translated from a future of wasted time into a future of prospects and anticipation. Once it becomes apparent that the world of mental handicap is on a different time line, we begin to ask different questions, then to develop different temporal expectations.

A timetable which allows for the expression of the unexpected, the dynamic and the unpredictable by mentally handicapped people will help them become the masters, not the victims of time and assist them in the quest for competence, creativity and community. As we have noted, for some mentally handicapped persons, time is an enemy. Getting through the day in the institution, or getting people out of the house to the day centre become aims in themselves. Apathetic staff and bored users stagnate together. This book has tried to explain that this is not inevitable. In describing the conscious pursuit of time, if only from Monday to Friday, this book has shown that time can be an ally, that the clock can enlarge the boundaries of routine, that competence, creativity and community can master time and not the reverse.

Potentially, this book could relate to a wider group than those who are mentally handicapped – its concepts might apply just as readily to the elderly, to unemployed young people, or to the physically and mentally disabled. In a changing society where full-time paid employment can no longer be viewed as the unquestioned norm of the future, mentally handicapped persons could be pioneers of a new use of time, for a future form of social life based on personal and social development through the tasks of group living.

By demonstrating that time is not always about money, that time is not always about paid work, mentally handicapped people may have statements to make to the rest of us. In a world with an increasing use of leisure time, people whose lives are not bounded by the factory whistle or the office deadline have things to teach the rest of us about the constructive use of leisure.

With this in mind, we can return to our initial questions and ask whether or not it is possible to foster and develop competence, creativity and community in settings for mentally handicapped people. To take competence first: the book has demonstrated how it was possible for some mentally handicapped people to begin to solve their everyday and future problems. A repertoire of ways of using time to do this has been outlined. It appears from our evidence that competence develops in settings in which individual objectives are quite highly specified over time, but where those concerned have some say over the content of their programmes of activities and a choice over the possible range of activities. Further, we saw that the aims for each user were described in clear, everyday language and that reviews were specified at certain time periods.

Priestley and his colleagues, in their book *Social Skills and Personal Problem Solving* (1978) described a series of similar assumptions which underpin the development of a sense of competence, and amplify the practices discussed in this book. He lists the importance of common sense; the process of coming to define a problem oneself, voluntarily; the necessity of variety and choice; the need for explicit language; the importance of openness by staff; the need for equality in relationships between staff and users; a belief in optimism and cheerfulness. All these issues have been discussed in previous chapters as fundamental conditions to developing competence. To take Dee as an example, we noted the importance of *assessment*, in the sense of defining both her difficulties and assets in as much detail as possible, in order to go on to set practical *objectives*. *Methods of learning* were specified and practised again and again, within everyday situations. We saw the failure of rapport with her home. Then we noted that regular *evaluations* check on progress and provide feedback, so that it is possible to decide whether to or not to continue a method with her, to stop, or to try something else. So the progressive development of competence was feasible in the right environment, given the appropriate time structures, the right attitudes and (probably least important) the up-to-date techniques.

What might be said about creativity? Recently there has been some discussion about the use of the arts for disabled people (Lord 1981). One intriguing quesiton raised by the imformation we have discussed is whether creativity, or imaginative inventiveness, is present in some mentally handicapped persons at least. The film *Stepping Out* showed a group of mentally handicapped persons from a residential home in Sydney displaying a dance performance at the Sydney Opera House with Aldo Genarro: one example of artistic responsiveness, imitation and imaginative inventiveness at work. Some prominent artists have become certain that it is possible to elicit creative responses from even severely mentally handicapped persons. The work of Malcolm Williamson, composer and Master of the Queen's Music, with severely mentally handicapped children and young adults suggests that it is possible for mentally handicapped people both to respond to music (to imitate and to perform it) and also to create it. In doing so Malcolm Williamson notes progress in the development of personal skills and relationships with others.

One problem about discussing creativity in mentally handicapped persons is deciding on the criteria which should be applied to their artistic work. A current debate in the arts concerns questions of standards: is excellence an arbitrary standard, imposed by a small elite on traditional art forms, such as opera, which are the purview of the well heeled? Or are there other standards which might lead to excellence outside this frame of reference? For example, is amateur street theatre which relates the arts to the problems of a particular black community necessarily less excellent than a performance of a new opera for the cognoscenti at the Royal Opera House? Excellence can be achieved in both performances, but the standards by which each performance should be judged should relate to the history and culture of art forms prized in each community: i.e. one performance is no more culturally significant than the other.

If this argument is applied to the use of arts for mentally handicapped people, it will be seen readily that the history and culture of such a unique group has been barely explored. The usual practice, that of judging mentally handicapped people as deviants from the standards of intelligentsia, may not be the only option. We have indicated that people such as Sam have their own way of life and particular experiences, which cannot be judged by reference to the standards of the wider society. So a more rigorous examination of achievement *within* the distinctive mental, emotional and cultural context of mental handicap may lead us, as a society, to defining mental handicap quite differently – perhaps as a preliterate, figurative and emotionally open subculture, with capacity to enrich the wider society. Original paintings and profound musical creation is now found to be produced by persons thought to be mentally handicapped at least as often as by the passengers on the omnibus to Clapham. Tim's print series on London buses is an exceptional example of originality and perception.

What about community? In recent years, a little has been written on the development of a sense of community in residential settings for the mentally handicapped. For example, in his book *Commitment and Growth* Jean Vanier tells the story of developing residential communities for mentally handicapped people known as L'Arche (Vanier

1979). These communities involve those 'handicapped' and 'normal' who wish to commit themselves to a communal way of life on a religious basis, living and working together in rural surroundings, pursuing a self-sufficient life with the idea of promoting personal growth and spiritual development of all.

Therapeutic communities are the technical form of this idea. After the Second World War, therapeutic communities for the mentally ill were developed in some psychiatric hospitals, in homes and hostels. The concept spread to services for almost all groups other than the mentally ill – children and offenders. However, there has been very little consideration about the extent to which forms of the therapeutic community might be an appropriate way of living daily with mental handicap in hospital, hostel and day centre. Various ways in which centres for the mentally handicapped can become more communal and less hierarchical have been outlined in this book. But as David Anderson points out in his book *Social Work and Mental Handicap* (1982) not everyone is willing to try. Working with people who are in pain from disability is fraught with chaos and despair, as staff build heavy defences against pain. Some of the traditional assumptions of the therapeutic community confront the pain and chaos in an open way, by using methods of democratic participation, by the group as a whole making the rules and by the confrontational type of relationships known as 'reality testing'.

Therapeutic communities are unusual in mental handicap services and they may never become commonplace, because they need staff strongly committed to their ideals and values. But the advantage of such centres is that they represent ideal or Utopian communities; small societies which seek to foster growth and eventually the maturity of those who live there, an antidote to the competitiveness, self-interest and individualism of the world. Certainly, as seen by Jean Vanier, the founder of L'Arche Communities, such ways of living bring growth and joy to the helpers as well as to the helped and the two groups grow closer together.

One important by-product of the adoption of the method of the therapeutic community – whether day or residential – is that such a community allows for the negotiation of the rights of users, as well as for their needs. And the types of duties and obligations can be spelled out and agreed, so that the users, as well as the staff, develop responsibilities to each other and to the service. Self-contained communities which aim to be self-sufficient are more common, for obvious reasons, in residential settings, but rarely in day settings has the notion of self-sufficiency and self-regulation been explored. Yet, if centres are to be in the position of sustaining the same group of people for a lifetime, should not some day communities, at least, be developing in the direction of self-sufficient, self-regulating services? A weekly club for the older people? A drop-in centre for mothers and children?

As we have seen, Highbury Grove Centre demonstrates that it *is* possible to begin to develop consciously the practice of rights and obligations within the context of a caring service. At Highbury Grove the assumption of obligations and duties for users relates to the progressive development of independence. Thus more responsibility is expected from Sam than Leanne. Sam is responsible for turning up punctually at a voluntary job for two days a week and for joining in the gardening project at the Centre. She is also responsible for behaving as a young adult, with consideration and care towards others. Yet Sam sees the obligations placed on her by the Centre as insufficient for her abilities and a limit on her rights. She longs to test her obligations as a citizen in the community.

This book has tried to emphasize that it is insufficient to develop programmes that deal solely with the *needs* of mentally handicapped people. Without a prior consideration of rights, needs can be subjectively interpreted, in the eye of the beholder rather than the recipient. The introductory chapter 'Beginnings', suggested that one distinguishing feature of public attitudes to the mentally handicapped was their acceptance or otherwise of their basic human rights and that consideration of human needs alone was an insufficient basis for providing services, because this places one group of people (the staff) in the powerful position of defining the requirements of other people (the users) without reference to their political and civil rights. It was argued that the needs-based approach gives those who define the needs the power to dominate those who are so defined. Whether it is the psychoanalyst who defines the needs of patients, white politicians who prescribe the needs of the black families, or in the case of the subject matter of this book, the health or social service professionals who define the needs of the mentally handicapped, definitions of need alone can be arbitrary and paternalistic, unless they are based on practices which accept the human rights of people to equal, just and fair treatment. But if the interpreters of needs so do in the context of a prior ascceptance of rights, they will be concerned, inevitably, about questions of power and its checks and balances whilst they try to redress the imbalances in favour of the relatively powerless, in this case mentally handicapped individuals.

It is not, however, the purpose of this book to provide this analysis of the relationship between power, rights and needs as they relate to mentally handicapped people. A brief commentary is provided in Appendix I, but such a study awaits further research.

This book proposes one type of agenda for the time of mentally handicapped people which might be developed from now until the end of the century. It suggests that one priority is to develop places not so much where people are cared for, as where their needs are individualized and their rights given expression. In particular, Highbury Grove Centre in all its purpose, variety and colour has demonstrated that:

For everything, there is a season, and a time . . .
A time to be born, and a time to die;
a time to plant and a time to pluck . . .
A time to kill, and a time to heal;

a time to break down, and a time to build up;
a time to weep, and a time to laugh;
a time to mourn, and a time to dance . . .
a time to embrace, and a time to refrain from embracing;
a time to seek, and a time to lose;
a time to keep, and a time to cast away;
a time to rend and a time to sew
a time to keep silence, and a time to speak;
a time to love, and a time to hate;
a time for war, and a time for peace.

(Ecclesiastes 3: 1–8)

# Appendix I: Needs and Rights

We have discussed the everyday life of Highbury Grove Centre to illustrate that the practice of considering needs alone, and as of more importance than rights, can be one type of the less-than-human perspective. On the other hand, those concerned with the needs of mentally handicapped people (and this includes most professional groups – doctors, social workers, nurses and psychologists) might argue that it is unrealistic to implement political and civil rights for those with mental handicap, when they need special protection from the law on the grounds that they lack the full capacity of 'normal' adults.

To what extent, then, is there a conflict between the achievement of full civil rights for mentally handicapped people and their needs for special protection? Certainly it is common to find that both are promoted together: the right to be treated 'normally' as well as the need for special services and special treatment. The Declaration of the Rights of Disabled People (1975) by the United Nations (para. 3) says of disabled people:

whatever the origin, nature and seriousness of their handicap and disabilities . . . have the same fundamental rights as their fellow citizens of the same age, which implies first and foremost the right to enjoy a decent life, as normal and full as possible.

Then the Declaration spells out the rights of disabled people to civil and political liberties to medical care, to education and training, to a decent level of living, to a 'normal' living environment, within a family if possible, to participation in social and recreational facilities, and to protection from exploitation, abuse or degradation.

So on the one hand, the Declaration implies that mentally handicapped people are to have access to the rights of every adult – what we might call 'general' rights (Houlgate 1980). Yet at the same time, the contradiction is that those who argue for 'general' rights also wish to promote 'special' rights for mentally handicapped people, such as special protection (the rights not to be abused, degraded or exploited), the claims to special services which enable them to enjoy access to the general rights listed above. The argument for 'rights' is complex because it involves the provision of special treatment and protection in order to be 'normal' and thereby to make proper use of general rights.

One of the key difficulties for those who wish to promote reforms for mentally handicapped people is to achieve a balance, or ratio between these two aspects of rights, the general and the special. In a climate where there are those who favour expenditure cuts on social services, pursuing the general right of 'normality' may be attractive, because it offers authorities the opportunity to defer the implementation of 'special' rights to special services which require extra levels of spending.

The argument, then, for rights for mentally handicapped people is complex. It requires 'special' rights to go in tandem with 'general' rights. The policy issue is what balance of either is appropriate at a given time. The pursuit of general rights is likely to be at the expense of special rights and vice versa. This leads either to an overdevelopment of special services and a lack of political and civil rights for the mentally handicapped; or to a consensus about political rights, but an absence of the special services required as means to the end of achieving full human status.

There is a further problem: whose responsibility is it to implement the rights of mentally handicapped persons? If there are rights, there are also claims. So if mentally handicapped adults have special and general rights, on whom or on what can handicapped persons make claims? A *child* who is mentally handicapped has some restricted claims on parents in children's law, as, of course, have those children who are not mentally handicapped. But when mentally handicapped children become adults with rights, on whom can they claim? Can parents be held to be responsible to implement their child's rights after their handicapped child reaches adulthood? Many accept this as a duty, but others do not or cannot. Should the state accept the legal responsibility of being the duty bearer? For example, should mentally handicapped adults be able to make individual claims on the state for rights to housing, education, social security, employment and medical services?

In Britain, the Chronically Sick and Disabled Persons Act 1970 was initial legislation which specified some particular claims that an adult handicapped person may make on the state. But the Act is really geared to definitions of physical handicap; the claims are highly restricted; and the obligations of authorities are permissive and voluntary, with no penalties against inaction. Whereas parents who do not meet the minimal legal standards prescribed to meet the claims of their children can be prosecuted under criminal law or taken before a juvenile court under civil law, no similar mechanism exists for the adult mentally handicapped person to pursue claims against public authorities.

So, at present, there is little to back up the rights of adult mentally handicapped persons to a decent life other than the goodwill of governments and authorities, the vocational commitment of the professional community and the moral fervour of pressure groups. And now, when public goodwill towards its disadvantaged members is in shorter supply, there is nothing to stop any social gains achieved for the rights of adult mentally handicapped persons being reversed. It is plain to see that the needs of the mentally handicapped are easier to meet than their rights. The definition of needs can be an arbitrary, selective, one-off exercise subject to cultural definition, relative, fragile and impermanent. Meeting needs is altogether less problematic than implementing, in tandem, special and general rights. But in Victoria, Australia, the State Government introduced legislation in 1987 to set up a Guardianship Board and a Guardianship Tribunal to protect the special rights of intellectually handicapped and other handicapped people in that State. These initiatives are an attempt to acknowledge the 'special' aspects of rights for handicapped people with the general rights of all citizens.

# Appendix II:
# Personal Assessment Sheet

| | | Dates of Assessment | | | | | |
|---|---|---|---|---|---|---|---|
| **A** | **Body Function** | | | | | | |
| 1 | Toilets self (day). | | | | | | |
| 2 | Toilets self (night). | | | | | | |
| 3 | Feeds self. | | | | | | |
| 4 | Washes self regularly. | | | | | | |
| 5 | Cleans own teeth regularly. | | | | | | |
| 6 | Bathes/showers self regularly. | | | | | | |
| 7 | (a) (man) Shaves when necessary. (b) (woman) Understands and copes with menstruation. (Cycle, disposal of sanitary towels, etc.) | | | | | | |

Key ✔ Does Without Prompting
  ○ Does With Prompting
  * High Priority Goal
  + Low Priority Goal
  – Not Allowable Goal

Dates of Assessment

| | | | | | | |
|---|---|---|---|---|---|---|
| 8  Understands the importance of personal hygiene. | | | | | | |
| 9  Knows basic dietary rules. (Regularity, types of food, etc.) | | | | | | |
| 10  Is able to discipline self *re* intake of appropriate food. | | | | | | |
| 11  Takes adequate exercise. | | | | | | |
| 12  Reacts appropriately to body signals; e.g. over-exertion, headache, toilet, etc. | | | | | | |
| 13  Uses basic first aid. | | | | | | |
| 14  Contacts doctors/hospital/ dentist if necessary. | | | | | | |
| 15  Seeks appropriate assistance for any of the above. | | | | | | |
| 16  Is aware of own sexuality (gender). | | | | | | |
| 17  Is aware of implications of male/female relationship (sexual and other). | | | | | | |
| 18  Knows basic facts of life (intercourse and result). | | | | | | |
| 19  Is aware of function and means of contraception. | | | | | | |
| 20  Seeks assistance for contraceptive advice and supply. | | | | | | |

Dates of Assessment

| | | | | | | |
|---|---|---|---|---|---|---|
| 21 | Is appropriately modest. | | | | | |
| 22 | Knows basic child care procedures. | | | | | |
| 23 | Cares independently for a child. | | | | | |
| 24 | Is aware of effects of age on body function. (Menopause, deterioration of tissues, etc.) | | | | | |
| 25 | Is aware of own physical handicap (if any). | | | | | |
| **B** | **Body Movement and Communication** | | | | | |
| 1 | Is aware of own identity (personal characteristics and information). | | | | | |
| 2 | Reacts appropriately to other individuals in relation to self. | | | | | |
| 3 | In communication, makes appropriate use of<br>i eye contact;<br>ii facial expression;<br>iii gesture. | | | | | |
| 4 | Understands non-verbal cues relating to initiation and termination of social contacts. | | | | | |
| 5 | Communicates needs/wants<br>i verbally;<br>ii non-verbally. | | | | | |

Dates of Assessment

| | | | | | |
|---|---|---|---|---|---|
| 6  Responds to communication<br> i verbally;<br> ii non-verbally. | | | | | |
| 7  Responds to rational discussion and argument. | | | | | |
| 8  Instigates rational discussion and argument. | | | | | |
| 9  Uses language creatively and imaginatively. | | | | | |
| 10  Has realistic self image<br> i physical;<br> ii mental. | | | | | |
| 11  Has good control of movement<br> i gross motor;<br> ii fine motor. | | | | | |
| 12  Has good posture. | | | | | |
| 13  Has good control of body in<br> i sports;<br> ii dance;<br> iii according to environment. | | | | | |
| 14  Uses body imaginatively. | | | | | |
| **C  Dress and Care of Dress** | | | | | |
| 1  Dresses self in correct sequence. | | | | | |
| 2  Undresses self. | | | | | |

Dates of Assessment

| | | | | | | |
|---|---|---|---|---|---|---|
| 3 Chooses appropriate clothing (according to climate and occasion). | | | | | | |
| 4 Purchases clothing of correct size and suitable style. | | | | | | |
| 5 Changes clothes according to function, time and cleanliness. | | | | | | |
| 6 Discards clothes when appropriate. | | | | | | |
| 7 Mends clothes when appropriate. | | | | | | |
| 8 Washes clothes when appropriate. | | | | | | |
| 9 Irons clothes when appropriate. | | | | | | |
| 10 Understands the necessity of 3–9 above and seeks appropriate assistance. | | | | | | |
| **D Domestic Environment** | | | | | | |
| 1 Implements order within the environment (i.e. knows where to put things in order to be able to find them again). | | | | | | |
| 2 In domestic environment, understands gas and electricity supplies (meters, mains taps, switches, etc.). | | | | | | |

Dates of Assessment

| | | | | | | |
|---|---|---|---|---|---|---|
| 3 Understands and takes into account safety precautions with domestic equipment and power supplies (fire risks, dangers of water and electricity, changing light bulbs etc.). | | | | | | |
| 4 Knows who and how to contact in an emergency (doctor, gas, electricity, etc.). | | | | | | |
| 5 Has basic domestic skills (cleaning, bed-making, etc.). | | | | | | |
| 6 Has more complex domestic skills (use of domestic machinery). | | | | | | |
| 7 Seeks out community facilities unaided (launderette, PO, etc.). | | | | | | |
| 8 Is hygienic in handling of food. | | | | | | |
| 9 (a) Can prepare and serve simple beverage.<br>(b) Washes up and tidies away afterwards. | | | | | | |
| 10 (a) Can prepare and serve simple snack.<br>(b) As 9(b). | | | | | | |
| 11 (a) Can prepare and serve simple meal.<br>(b) As 9(b). | | | | | | |

Dates of Assessment

| | | | | | | |
|---|---|---|---|---|---|---|
| 12 | Can recognize and select appropriate utensils and packages for 9, 10, 11. | | | | | |
| 13 | Shops unaided for items. | | | | | |
| 14 | Has acceptable eating habits. | | | | | |
| 15 | Keeps cooking/eating environment clean and tidy. | | | | | |
| 16 | Recognizes and selects cleaning materials/ implements needed for 15. | | | | | |
| 17 | Shops unaided for items needed above. | | | | | |
| 18 | Travels alone (walking) locally. | | | | | |
| 19 | Travels alone (walking), more complex journeys. | | | | | |
| 20 | Travels short distances using public transport (bus, tube, etc.). | | | | | |
| 21 | Travels more complex journeys alone, using public transport (changing buses, combinations of bus/tube/walking, etc.). | | | | | |
| 22 | Travels to Centre alone by any of above. | | | | | |
| 23 | Understands the composition of the family group. | | | | | |

Dates of Assessment

| | | | | | | |
|---|---|---|---|---|---|---|
| 24  Understands and fulfils demands of family group. | | | | | | |
| 25  Participates in other forms of group living (group home, hostel). | | | | | | |
| 26  Fulfils requirements and demands of this group. | | | | | | |
| **E  Work** | | | | | | |
| 1  Understands the significance of work as a means of earning money in order to live. | | | | | | |
| 2  Understands routine implicit in work (starting time, finishing time, breaks). | | | | | | |
| 3  Participates willingly in individual work. | | | | | | |
| 4  Participates willingly in group work. | | | | | | |
| 5  Has work outside the centre  i  paid;  ii voluntary. | | | | | | |
| 6  Completes simple new tasks (1 stage)  i  with supervision;  ii without supervision. | | | | | | |

Dates of Assessment

| | | | | | | |
|---|---|---|---|---|---|---|
| 7 | Completes relatively complex new tasks (5 stage)<br> i with supervision;<br>ii without supervision. | | | | | |
| 8 | Seeks help readily, if necessary. | | | | | |
| 9 | Accepts unsought help without expressing resentment. | | | | | |
| 10 | Understands his/her role in the team. | | | | | |
| 11 | Recognizes the role of others in the team. | | | | | |
| 12 | Recognizes and rectifies mistakes by self. | | | | | |
| 13 | Recognizes and points out mistakes by others in the team. | | | | | |
| 14 | Has realistic attitude to own work ability (including aspirations). | | | | | |
| **F** | **Pre-reading, Reading, Writing** | | | | | |
| 1 | Has good pre-reading skills. | | | | | |
| 2 | Is aware of the relevance of reading ability. | | | | | |

Dates of Assessment

| | | | | | |
|---|---|---|---|---|---|
| **3** Knows letters of the alphabet<br>  i by name;<br>  ii phonetically. | | | | | |
| **4** Has basic sight vocabulary<br>  i stage 1;<br>  ii stage 2;<br>  iii stage 3. | | | | | |
| **5** Reads well (simple new words using 3.ii). | | | | | |
| **6** Reads to obtain information. | | | | | |
| **7** Reads for pleasure (and comprehends). | | | | | |
| **8** Uses the library. | | | | | |
| **9** Writes own name:<br>  i prints;<br>  ii signs. | | | | | |
| **10** Fills in forms. | | | | | |
| **11** Communications in writing (letters, postcards, etc.). | | | | | |
| **12** Writes creatively and imaginatively. | | | | | |
| **G Number** | | | | | |
| **1** Can count and identify numbers 1–10. | | | | | |
| **2** Can count and identify all numbers. | | | | | |

Dates of Assessment

| | | | | | | |
|---|---|---|---|---|---|---|
| 3 Can count efficiently in practical situations<br>  i up to 10 times;<br> ii any number of items. | | | | | | |
| 4 Tells the time. | | | | | | |
| 5 Understands time in relation to the day's events. | | | | | | |
| 6 Understands time in relation to events of a longer duration. | | | | | | |
| 7 Plans use of time in daily needs. | | | | | | |
| 8 Understands and uses money. | | | | | | |
| 9 Looks after own money. | | | | | | |
| 10 Can budget<br>  i daily;<br> ii weekly;<br> iii long-term. | | | | | | |
| 11 Has a realistic and practical attitude towards money. | | | | | | |
| 12 Budgets for bills, HP, etc. | | | | | | |
| 13 Can calculate mentally (adding)<br>  i up to 10p;<br> ii up to 50p;<br> iii up to £1;<br> iv for any amount. | | | | | | |

Dates of Assessment

| | | | | | | |
|---|---|---|---|---|---|---|
| 14 Can calculate mentally (subtracting)<br>  i up to 10p;<br>  ii up to 50p;<br>  iii up to £1;<br>  iv for any amount. | | | | | | |
| 15 Saves<br>  i for specific plans;<br>  ii without definite target. | | | | | | |
| 16 Understands social implications of money (i.e. lending borrowing, stealing). | | | | | | |
| 17 Understands the more complex financial matters of tax, Nat. Insurance, etc. | | | | | | |
| 18 (a) Claims and cashes benefits.<br>(b) Understands mechanics of above. | | | | | | |
| 19 Understands various ways of saving (bank, PO, Building Society, etc.). | | | | | | |
| 20 Understands relevance and use of measurement (length, width, etc.). | | | | | | |
| 21 Uses ruler, tape measure correctly. | | | | | | |
| 22 Knows own sizes. | | | | | | |

Dates of Assessment

| | | | | | | |
|---|---|---|---|---|---|---|
| 23 Uses scales in<br>  i kitchen;<br> ii bathroom. | | | | | | |
| 24 Uses weight as<br>classification in<br>  i shopping;<br> ii recipes. | | | | | | |

# References

Anderson, D. (1982) *Social Work and Mental Handicap* (Macmillan, London).

Carter, J. (1981) *Day Services for Adults; Somewhere to Go* (George Allen and Unwin, London).

Cook, D. (1981) *Winter Doves* (Penguin, Harmondsworth).

Houlgate, H. (1980) *The Child and the State: A Normative Theory of Juvenile Rights* (Johns Hopkins University Press, Baltimore).

Jones, K. (1975) *Opening the Door; Study of New Policies for the Mentally Retarded* (Routledge and Kegan Paul, London).

King, R., Raynes, N. and Tizard, J. (1971) *Patterns of Residential Care* (Routledge and Kegan Paul, London).

Lane, H. (1977) *The Wild Boy of Aveyron* (George Allen and Unwin, London).

Lord, G. (1981) *The Arts and Disabilities: a Creative Response to Social Handicap* (Macdonald Publishers, Edinburgh).

MacLean, C. (1979) *The Wolf Children* (Penguin, Harmondsworth).

Mittler, P. (1979) *People, Not Patients; Problems and Policies in Mental Handicap* (Methuen, London).

Priestley, P., McGuire, J., Flegg, D., Hemsley, V. and Welham, D. (1978) *Social Skills and Personal Problem Solving* (Tavistock, London).

Raynes, N.V., Pratt, M. and Roses, S.R. (1979) *Organisational Structure and the Care of the Mentally Retarded* (Croom Helm, London).

Ryan, J. (1980) *The Politics of Mental Handicap* (Penguin, Harmondsworth).

Strauss, A. and Glaser, B. (1977) *Anguish: A Case History of a Dying Trajectory* (Martin Robertson, London).

Vanier, J. (1979) *Commitment and Growth* (St. Paul Publications, Sydney).